Praise for *FibroWHYalgia*....

"Millions suffer with fibromyalgia and can benefit from the detailed and practical resource guide that Susan Ingebretson has compiled. Carefully following her advice will go a long way toward helping resolve this illness, which is particularly resistant to most conventional treatments that fail to incorporate the valuable principles described in this book."

Dr. Joseph Mercola, Founder, http://www.Mercola.com/
the world's most visited natural health site
Hoffman Estates, Illinois

"I absolutely love this informative book! Susan Ingebretson's humor and insight make *FibroWHYalgia* a 'page turner' and a delight to read. Filled with valuable lessons, this book is for EVERYONE — those with ailments and those interested in preventing them."

Linda J. Miner, RNC, CHN, RSNA, CMTA, BA
nutritional expert, wellness guide, Creator of
http://www.MyHealthyBalance.com/
and http://www.iChange.com/
British Columbia, Canada

"*FibroWHYalgia* doesn't pretend to have all the answers but does offer smart solutions helpful to anyone wishing to kick-start a wellness plan. I love the combination of Midwestern wit and common sense used to deliver the message of healing. If you're sick and tired of being sick and tired, the upbeat suggestions in this book will provide the encouragement needed to seek positive change."

Mollie Marti, PhD, JD
Performance psychologist and Creator of
http://www.BestLifeDesign.com/
Cedar Rapids, Iowa

"As a practitioner specializing in chronic conditions, I consider *FibroWHYalgia* a first-aid kit for anyone dealing with long-term health issues. The tools needed to rebuild wellness are laid out in an easy-to-understand style that's entertaining to read. I stock this book in my store and offer it as recommended reading to my patients."

Diane Wendell, ND, CNM, nutritionist
http://www.ShopNutritionPlus.com/
Tustin, California

"*FibroWHYalgia* simplifies the underlying physiology of fibromyalgia. Readers will come away armed with an understanding of why they might have this or another chronic condition and with lifestyle strategies to navigate from illness to wellness. What I loved most about this delightful book is Susan Ingebretson's determination, wit, and resilience to find answers to heal herself—despite a medical system that provides little hope."

C. Jessie Jones, PhD, professor, Health Science
Director, Fibromyalgia Research and Education Center
California State University, Fullerton

"Reading *FibroWHYalgia* was like stepping out of a cold fog into the warm sun. Susan Ingebretson cuts through the confusing muddle of fibromyalgia information and misinformation, providing factual encouragement that *anyone* can put into practice. This book is for anyone touched by fibromyalgia or other chronic illness. Because this encouraging, humor-filled book is backed by science and real-life experience, every chronic illness support group should have copies of this book available for its members. I keep multiple copies in my practice's lending library."

Pamela Reilly, CNHP, CPH
Naturopath, Living Foods Life Coach,
http://www.GoodWorksWellness.com/
Indianapolis, Indiana

"*FibroWHYalgia,* written in a humorous and friendly style, is seasoned with wit, wisdom, and encouragement. It's an easy-to-read, non-technical guide for those suffering from chronic illness. As a certified holistic health and nutrition counselor, I'm pleased to find tips and ideas on how to maintain a healthy lifestyle. Susan Ingebretson's unique 'Ten Roots to a Better You' section provides healing practitioners such as nutritionists, chiropractors, personal trainers, etc., with a useful tool for their clients."

Irina Wardas, CHHC
Holistic Health and Wellness Services for Women
http://www.NaturalCounselor.com/
Carlsbad, California

"Like a roadmap, *FibroWHYalgia* points the way toward healing for both the newly diagnosed and the long-term chronic illness patient."

Timothy Noble, DC, DACBSP, CSCS
http://www.AnaheimHillsChiropractic.com/
Anaheim Hills, California

"*FibroWHYalgia* is clear, practical, and enjoyable. In a style like a comfortable conversation with a friend, Susan Ingebretson leads us down her path of self-discovery and encourages us to take responsibility for our own health through essential lifestyle changes. If you're ready for a change, this is the book for you. The chapter on nutrition is the most sensible and concise information I've found and is a must-read, chronically ill or not. Through her hard-fought battle to understand the root causes of her symptoms and her determined journey to recover, Susan Ingebretson proves wellness is an option."

Dannette Mason Rusnak, Creator of
FibroHaven Support Foundation
http://www.FibroHaven.com/
Carlsbad, California

for my sisters

FibroWHYalgia

Why REBUILDING the
Ten Root Causes of Chronic Illness
RESTORES Chronic Wellness

Susan E. Ingebretson

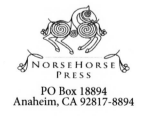

NORSEHORSE
PRESS

PO Box 18894
Anaheim, CA 92817-8894

WARNING AND DISCLAIMER: The information herein is not intended to diagnose, treat, cure, or prevent any disease, nor has this material been evaluated by the Food and Drug Administration. All information relating to medical conditions, health issues, products, and treatments are not meant to be a substitute for the advice of your own physician or other medical professional. You should not use the information herein to diagnose or treat yourself and should consult with your physician or medical professional before making changes to medications or doctor-recommended programs of any kind.

ISBN: 978-0-9843118-0-4

Library of Congress Control Number: 2009943569

Printed in the United States of America

Ordering information: http://www.rebuildingwellness.com/

NorseHorse Press
PO Box 18894
Anaheim, CA 92817-8894

Contents

Preface

Can a cup of tea and a tenacious personality conquer chronic illness? For me, yes. When I realized that my body was failing, I had to know why.

Armed with tea and my laptop, I scoured online medical articles, white papers, journals, and newsletters. I obtained enough books to seed an acre of ideas.

Notes jotted onto spiral-bound pages became the basis for ongoing research, processing, reference, and this book. But not every jot and tittle of research is included, just the high spots. It's as simple as this: I did my homework.

Fibromyalgia is my diagnosis, and these contents reflect my personal experiences. However, the hints, helps, and histories apply to anyone pursuing better health and striving to capture wellness.

I have inserted tea tag witticisms and quotes throughout this book. The relationship between tea and health is both entertaining and educational. Tea tags are the philosophical MFA program for the armchair set.

So, pour a steaming cup and read on.

*Think of the following
as pearls of wisdom
knotted together into an elegant,
painted macaroni necklace.*

Introduction

The workings of the brain fascinate me. While giving a speech on health and nutrition in a hospital auditorium, someone in the audience caught my eye. As I observed her movements, my brain simultaneously directed my mouth to form the words of my presentation while other thoughts and ideas continued to spin. My gaze bounced between the audience and my candy-colored note cards. Aware that I appeared single-focused, I knew I was not.

My thoughts wandered. How could I speak and observe at the same time? How does the brain do that? Wait a minute! That's three things: I was talking, observing, *and* analyzing.

The brain is fascinating. I'm especially intrigued, knowing that mine is damaged and prone to information misfires, but we'll get to that later.

During my lecture, the faint odor of disinfectant wafted through the auditorium; my eyes watered. I blinked but couldn't resist staring at the woman in the audience. Her pen swept over the handout where I'd provided a tight ladder of lines for notes. Large letters angled across the page. Her tongue peeked from her lips in concentration. With a final flourish, she stabbed her comment with a squadron of punctuation.

What did I say to cause such a response? I felt my shoulders rise, my spine straighten. Question & Answer time arrived. Surely, she would raise her hand first.

Nope.

I continued to answer questions and maneuvered toward the back of the auditorium. I positioned myself to glance casually over her shoulder to read the scrawled note.

This attendee summarized my thirty-minute speech in three larger-than-life words: EAT GOOD CHOCOLATE!!!

"*To know the road ahead, ask those coming back.*"

—Chinese Proverb

Chapter 1

The Genesis of a Hypothesis

My quest for wellness has been a long one. I've learned that my past has more to do with my present than I thought possible. I've learned to research, review, and respect my cultural and genetic heritage — the foundation of who I am.

The following scenarios offer insight into why I call myself a "slow boil," and how my heritage helped open the door to chronic illness.

To see the future, I looked back. History repeats itself. Analysis of the past provided dependable predictions for my future. Taking a personal inventory of my heritage and characteristics of my ancestors revealed more about me than I expected.

I grew up in rural Iowa, a land where tornadoes propel weeds through tree trunks, shoreless seas fall from the sky, and burly snow drifts camouflage fences from October through April.

Factor into this inhospitable environment, the people. Like so many contradictions of nature, Iowa is populated with the friendliest folk this side of Greece. Kind, hard-working, and polite enough to annoy a New Yorker at ten paces.

Many of these Iowans are Scandinavians (Norse, Swedes, and Danes). Combine Scandinavian and Midwestern traits and what do you get? A farmer who'd selflessly feed a passel of strangers but hasn't spoken to his own brother (on the acreage next door) in over thirty years. Stubbornness runs in the genes and the overalls.

A magnet on my fridge reads: *You can always tell a Norwegian … but you can't tell him much.* I've often thought mules and Norwegians have much in common, and some ancestral tintype photos seem to support my theory.

In addition to stubborn, "stoic" is an apt description of Midwestern Scandinavians. They're as demonstrative as the Queen Mum and her cheery family. The emotion of the famous Grant Wood painting is spot on. It's officially titled, "American Gothic: Oil on Beaverboard." You can't get more Midwestern than that.

The portrait of my heritage is pretty clear. It's no cosmic fluke that I spent a lifetime working hard, burning the candle at both ends, putting my needs last. Add injury and traumatic stress to that mix, and physical illness was a statistical probability. Just as predictable was my slow response to my physical breakdown.

I make better choices now.

⁂

This was the genesis of my hypothesis. Remember the science experiment with frogs and boiling water? I wrote the name "Stu" under the frog's picture in my high school textbook. To review, a living frog can be slowly boiled to death when placed in a pot of water over steadily increasing heat. The point being, even though it *can* jump out of the pot, it *doesn't*.

It's my hypothesis that Norwegians under pressure are the human equivalent of those frogs.

Some differences are obvious, such as skin color and habitat. Other differences, not so. Norwegians aren't likely to jump in excitement, anger, or happiness. Barring flames coming from their shoes, Norwegians don't jump at all. Emotions are displayed in cryptic, subtle cues.

> One raised eyebrow = surprise
> Two raised eyebrows = great excitement or joy
> Two raised eyebrows and, "I might call 9-1-1"
> = extreme panic or alarm

I think of the frog's inaction as contentment rather than a lack of intelligence. Maybe frogs are happy where they are? Well, frogs may be victims of their genetics, but we don't have to be. We can take action. Someday, we may even jump from the pot.

The comparison between Norwegians and laboratory frogs that don't jump out of the hot water is familiar for many. We often ignore what's really going on, focusing instead on the inside of the pot. Meanwhile, the surrounding temperature rises dangerously from bath to broth. It's tough to recognize when we need to take that lifesaving leap.

My dad often repeated a story about our ancestors. Fed up with the conditions of their icy homelands, early Scandinavians sailed to America packed in boats like King Oscar Sardines. They traversed prairies in crude wagons and survived the perils of the "Mighty Mississip" only to make the upper Midwest their home — a land just as frozen and forsaken as the one they left behind!

The only appropriate response to that story is, "*uff-da*," a Scandinavian expression that's a cross between Piglet's "Oh d-d-dear, dear" and Frank Barone's "Holy crap!" (from *Everybody Loves Raymond*).

> "*Unless we change our direction, we're likely to end up where we are headed.*"
> —Chinese Proverb

When my grandmother spilled coins from her purse, she muttered, "*uff-da*." When a drunk driver plowed his Buick into her pumpkin-colored house, her "*UFF-da!*" went up an octave.

As in so much of life, *how* you say it makes all the difference.

Influenced by my heritage and environment, my personality traits morphed into the beginnings of "me."

Iowa in the 1970s exemplified a simpler time, but it was not carefree. In rural areas, agricultural pesticides were sprayed freely, with little care. Chemicals permeated the air and seeped into our underground wells. Straight from the tap, we drank carrot-colored water with black and grey flecks. No one seemed to care.

I often visited my friends' rural homes. Iowa farmers are a hardy bunch. From inside the house, I watched them spray crops and learned that real men don't wear protective face masks. I was told that insecticides were harmless to people and killed "just the bugs." It sounded like a fair swap to me: a little stink for no bugs.

Through the family room window, I remember seeing bare-faced men spraying the fields. Noxious clouds reached the house, stinging my eyes. I threw my arm over my face, my nose tucked in the crook of my elbow, as I heard a perfume jingle on TV, "*Her Windsong stays on my mind...*"

Looking back, I can pinpoint many experiences that may have negatively impacted my health. Chronic illness travels a slow and twisted path. It would be nice to find a single, culpable source (even better, one with deep pockets), but that's unlikely.

Those who kick up the dust of their pasts will probably be able to recognize an assortment of environmental co-factors that could have contributed to their eventual impaired health. By linking them together, individual historical health chains can be revealed.

Past experiences color our current perceptions. To this day, many perfumes smell like DDT to me.

℘

Tenth grade year: We were all abuzz over our American history project. A handout received several months prior outlined the simple requirements: read a book; write a paper. But, this was a big to-do — footnotes, bibliography, the works.

There were ten book options, from thick to thin. Most of my classmates chose the first book, *PT 109*, with two-hundred pages. I slogged through *Armageddon*, from the bottom of the list, just shy of eight-hundred pages.

As a burgeoning history buff, I loved the book. I sweated over the writing assignment. No one was more surprised than I to discover I had something to say.

I passed in my report, the transparent cover bent under the weight. On the teacher's desk, it looked out of place stacked with the other wispy offerings. I hoped for an A; I dreamed of a plus next to it.

When the time came, my teacher, a grim football coach with a stereotypical butch haircut, black-framed glasses, and bulldog underbite, called me to the front of the classroom. He handed me my report, and I saw the plus. Everything I'd dreamed of! But he snarled, "You didn't write this."

I looked again. There was a plus sign, but no A. I saw a D-plus.

My face felt hot. "You don't talk like this, so you couldn't write like this," he said. I went back to my seat in stony silence.

I can think of many retorts, now. *From what source would I plagiarize? Who says verbal skills equate to writing skills?* A shy student, I rarely spoke in class. How he drew his conclusion I'll never know. Aptly named, my *Armageddon* experience snuffed out my budding writer's voice without a whimper.

There's an important lesson here exposing a secondary characteristic of mine. The most telling part of this tale was not my passive behavior. Nope. The most revealing tidbit is tucked near the beginning. What book did I select? I went for the most difficult of all. Given the choice between easy and difficult, there was no middle road for me. This trait has dominated my life's decisions; I have yet to choose an easy path.

Like many Scandinavians, I distrust my own feelings. I wonder, *do I really feel that?* Or, *what is that niggling worry in my chest?*

Inner dialogue is an energy-zapper. Fatigued by second-guessing myself, I'm too tired to take on anyone else. I am a "slow boil," and I willingly pin the blame on my heritage. Relatives stick together, sharing the common bond of family history and finger-pointing.

In real life, action and reaction don't happen as on TV. Actors show instant access to emotions, but for others, this access may be delayed.

Consider the Sunday I weeded my front yard with Foxy, my nine-pound Sheltie, on duty (barking at nefarious crows). A stranger jogged up the opposite side of the street, pulled by a huge German shepherd. Foxy took off in pursuit before I could blink. Flapping her arms at both dogs, the stranger keened like an island native at a chieftain's funeral.

A minute later, Foxy was back at my side, leaving the stranger to sprint downhill — still wailing. I picked up my pup and scolded her for un-neighborly behavior. Her face was wet, her eyes swollen. Then, I smelled it.

The stranger had pepper-sprayed my dog!

I immediately washed her face and took her to the groomers. The receptionist asked if Foxy had jumped on or bitten the stranger. No. So why the pepper spray? Furious that someone had hurt such a little mop of a dog, she asked if I was mad, too.

Mad … *moi?*

My only feeling was guilt over Foxy's misbehavior. I went door to door to see if my neighbors knew the stranger. I wanted to apologize. As I retold the story, finding that my neighbors agreed with the receptionist surprised me.

My guilt ebbed as anger finally began to flow. The stranger *could* have used other tactics, right? I played the scene over in my mind, remembering the German shepherd looking bored while the woman screamed. Who was the hysterical party?

By Monday, I simmered. News spread and concerned neighbors asked about Foxy. I was glad to report a full recovery. By Wednesday, I was downright ticked off. The temperature in my pot had finally reached boiling.

> "*You cannot teach a man anything; you can only help him find it within himself.*"
>
> —Galileo Galilei

I gained two lessons from this experience (three, if you count learning how to rinse pepper spray from a dog's eyes). First, it took four days for me to recognize how I felt; second, it took the nudging of others to get me there. It's a good thing nothing vital hung in the balance while the world waited for my opinion.

This episode illustrates how I can be smart and dumb at the same time. I'm quick-witted, yet slow to act. I possess aptitude and skill, but I distrust my ability to put them into action.

Now you know why it took not years but *decades* to figure out my health issues. Yes, I'm a slow boil, and that's what nearly killed me!

"Trust thyself only,
and another shall
not betray thee."

—Thomas Fuller

Chapter 2

Diagnosis: The Sequins of Events

Chronic illness creeps up slowly; it took ages for me to accept that I was truly ill. Finding the appropriate diagnosis took just as long and became my Holy Grail. I sought answers with zeal, navigating the maze of tests and scans, looking for *the* answer — the correct diagnosis. As it happened, I had to figure it out for myself. Then, I had to determine what that diagnosis meant.

In my mid-thirties, I watched my health spiral out of control. I was achy, nauseous, and dizzy. Raging intestinal troubles squelched personal freedoms. Believing I had contracted a nasty bug on a mission trip to Mexico, I went for blood tests. Dr. X speculated that parasites had taken up residence in my intestines.

Finding none, Dr. X declared me well. I didn't feel well. "Wait it out," he said. "You'll be fine."

I did. But I was not.

Weeks dragged, and so did I. The pain and fatigue grew. I set my alarm earlier each day to compensate for increased morning sluggishness. Getting out of bed took gargantuan effort. I grasped my heavy nightstand for support and inched my legs to the side of the mattress. Swinging them to the floor, I collapsed onto my knees, still holding the nightstand. Using the Lamaze method for pain management, I army-crawled to the bathroom. By the time my kids were awake, I was showered and quasi-vertical, though still in extreme pain. I was single and glad of it. Divorced at the time, I had no other adult to bear witness to this daily spectacle.

The fact remained: My body *betrayed* me. Muscles burned. Joints ached. Even my teeth hurt. My bones felt fractured and detached from ligaments and tendons. My digestive tract functioned like a sieve. My body's systems failed little by little.

Each day I regressed further toward incapacitation. My muscles were defective. What kind of bizarre disease was this? I could barely move, but necessary employment forced me to the office each day. By seven p.m., fatigue swallowed me whole, and I crawled into bed for another fitful night of no sleep.

Days blurred; summer arrived. It seemed as if a giant, Dijon-colored balloon was stretched over my head. A murky, yellow-brown veil cloaked my view of the world, my vision dimmed. My brain functioned in time-delayed motion. Removed by pain, I was aware of my surroundings, but only in a surreal way. Reality dangled vaguely out of reach.

I stood at death's door but lacked the strength to knock.

I saw Dr. X ten more times. On the morning of visit seven, a painful rash appeared across my chest. The skin burned as I scratched through my sequin-embellished T-shirt.

A snarky receptionist rolled her eyes when she called my name. "You can go back to Exam Room Three and … if you wanna know, your shirt's inside out."

I was a physical and emotional glob.

My equilibrium worsened; furniture and walls became my support systems. Eleventy-nine blood tests later, still no diagnosis. Nurses drew blood from the backs of my hands. My bruised inner forearms looked as if stained with fruity tattoos of plums and berries.

To soothe my intestinal tornado, I nibbled on bits of crackers and dry cereal. With so few calories, I should have shriveled to almost nothing. I did not. Instead, my body swelled — particularly my abdomen. My temperature (feverish or freezing) fluctuated along with my vision. Objects sharpened in focus only to disappear again into the familiar yellow-brown haze.

Dr. X welcomed my presence as eagerly as a plantar wart. At each visit, he clutched his clipboard, handed me a new prescription to "try," and declared me well. His friendly greetings turned tepid. He acted as if I were starving for attention. He was half-right — I was starving. At least, that's what Felicity told me. Had we not crossed paths, I'm convinced my situation would have worsened beyond repair.

I met this angel in a supermarket parking lot. I'd fallen (again) on the blacktop and lay there summoning the energy to move. The only thing missing from my silhouette was a chalk outline. I debated whether to fish three soup cans from under my car when a kind woman offered help. Preferring anonymity, I didn't respond. She persisted. Supporting my elbow, she brought me upright and looked me straight in the eye.

She surveyed my face, then looked down and brushed parking lot pebbles from my palms. She carefully inspected my hands and fingers, paying particular attention to my nails. Her concern felt as thorough as any exam I'd had.

"Have you seen a doctor?"

I nodded and explained that I'd been given a clean bill of health.

She lifted my chin, bringing my gaze to meet hers. "You tell that doctor you're sick. The whites of your eyes and the color of your skin show me your liver's not working worth a damn. Your hands and nails tell me even more. Are you eating? You're severely malnourished. I think your organs are shutting down. *Make your doctor listen!*"

> "*All God's angels come to us disguised.*"
> —Plato

My first glimmer of validation. Though I never saw her again, I think of her as an angel. I've named her Felicity for the pivotal role she played in encouraging me to seek answers.

ﬆ

Acting on Felicity's mandate, I revisited Dr. X. I stated I was not well and not getting better. He sighed and said there was nothing wrong with me. I was annoyed when he asked about my personal life. After prodding, I mentioned my stressful relationship with my ex-husband as well as work pressures. He wanted to hear more. We continued with a discussion of my boyfriend's chemo treatments. He showed mild interest. He asked about my adult daughter who worked in his favorite lunchtime restaurant. Upon hearing the news I'd soon be a grandmother, he exclaimed, "Ah-ha!"

His official diagnosis? "Fear."

Dr. X declared I was afraid of growing old. There you have it. My physical breakdown was a manifestation of that fear. He patted himself on the back for unraveling the complexities of my condition.

I was shocked and didn't know what to say. I knew Dr. X well. He'd been my physician and friend for years. Expecting gratitude for his official diagnosis, he appeared surprised at my silence.

Already sick and tired, now I was labelled "old," too. No closer to a diagnosis, I walked away, never to return.

ℬ

Needing a change of scenery, I planned a cross-country road trip to see landmarks, my family, and to attend a class reunion. The Grand Canyon, Petrified Forest, and Meteor Crater looked like foggy postcards from my car window. I was too fatigued to get out and look. I did, however, visit every rest stop across ten states. My reunion capped off the trip. My classmates glimpsed a bloated, jaundiced me.

I returned home feeling no better, but determined to "get on" with things. I decided my "disease" wasn't going to kill me, that feeling worse was impossible. Why see another doctor who'd only tell me nothing's wrong?

I accepted a life of chronic illness. My boyfriend accepted no such thing. Feeling human again after his own cancer treatment, he wanted me to get better, too. He dragged me to a chiropractor who promised health and vitality to sedentary office workers. Unconvinced but willing, I committed to frequent treatments. My strength rose in direct correlation to my bank account's descent.

As an investment into my future, I achieved improvement in my digestive health first. Over the next six months, health and vitality returned. Slowly I crawled, and then walked, back into my old life.

Chiropractic cured the disease I was told I didn't have. After a year or two of good health, that earlier experience seemed like a bad dream. I questioned my memory and decided I'd had a severe bout of the twenty-four *month* flu.

ℬ

Fast-forward about five years. I remarried and was knee-deep in major home renovations. Tired, stressed, and frustrated, I emptied kitchen cabinets and stacked loaded boxes into the garage. My husband and I lifted the final item, a heavy, butcher-block table. That's when I felt it. A searing pain ripped across my upper back and electrified my left shoulder. Trying not to vomit, I panted and did Lamaze breathing. My left arm throbbed along with my spine and shoulder. My husband wanted me to go to the emergency room, but I shook my head. I couldn't think beyond panting. No rash decisions for this Norwegian. My husband repeatedly asked me to lie down or get in the car.

"Wait," I said.

As with past injuries, I waited for things to improve. I tried to lie down but shooting pain in my chest catapulted me to my feet. Upright and vertical was the only tolerable position. I paced. The overall pain didn't lessen, but didn't worsen, either. It made no sense. I was positive I'd suffered an aortic tear or something dire, but how could that be? I was still conscious.

I paced all night. The next morning, my husband shook his head in frustration. I couldn't inhale deeply or lie down, but I wouldn't go to the hospital. Deductive reasoning said it couldn't be a heart attack or stroke; I was neither dead nor paralyzed. I didn't want to face another there's-nothing-wrong-with-you doctor, so I simply didn't.

After four days, I finally saw my chiropractor. She took x-rays and tried to help me. She deserved an A for effort, but couldn't bring me relief. Her patience wore thin after a few months, and she suggested I see my general practitioner. We were both frustrated with my lack of progress.

Stubborn, I waited a while longer. I ferried kids to school and went to work. Driving was a nightmare. I developed thick calluses on my hands from my death grip on the steering wheel. My hilly neighborhood became the bane of my existence. Uphill, I pulled on the wheel to hold my fragile spine off of the seatback, the pressure otherwise unbearable. Downhill was worse. It felt as if my spine thrust forward through my chest wall. The earth's gravitational pull seemed amplified just for me.

Frazzled, I finally saw an osteopath. I saw Dr. Y about four months after the "kitchen table incident." He sent me for x-rays and said I probably pinched a nerve. I explained that I could only doze between shooting pains while sitting upright in a chair. I could not lie down. He frowned; I don't think he believed me.

Who was I kidding? *I* didn't believe me.

I told Dr. Y it felt as if I had a bullet wedged just to the left of my spine, midway between hips and shoulders. An aurora borealis of pain spun out from there, leaving the tissues in my entire back feeling swollen, hot, tender. The pain spread to my extremities with the brunt of it on my left side. The only tangible clues were finger-like black smudges across the left side of my chest. The still-unexplained bruises lasted nearly a year.

Dr. Y referred me to cardiologists, orthopedists, rheumatologists, neurologists, and physical therapists. No answers.

The United States declared war, and I did, too. Dr. Y went into the reserves as troops invaded Iraq. A kind, wet-behind-the-ears intern took over in his absence. She asked about symptoms I felt were unimportant: irritable bowel, muscle cramps, hormone fluctuations, etc. Right away she said, "I think your constellation of symptoms is part of a bigger health problem. It looks connective tissue-related."

For the first time, I saw the reality of my declining health. I realized how bleak my future would be without intervention. The new intern encouraged me to pursue a diagnosis and pointed me in the direction of autoimmune-related conditions. I made a decision to seek ways to intentionally rebuild wellness. *It was time for change, time for taking charge.*

I no longer waited passively for referrals and appointments. I made phone calls, faxed requests, and monitored my results. I took over the administrative role I'd mistakenly assigned to the doctor's office staff. Following protocol, I took every medication prescribed (numbering in double digits). I battled with my insurance company. I fought for approvals of MRIs and brain scans. I filled notebooks with test results, pending referral requests, and copies of insurance forms. For two years, I sought specialists who could point me in the right direction. I hunted a diagnosis with the focus (and success) of Elmer Fudd hunting wabbits.

My intended destination was a diagnosis. I arrived at desperation instead. Clutching a rheumatologist's lab coat at one visit, I begged for answers. He rolled his eyes and said, "Just accept it. You'll never know what's wrong with you."

ℒ

With no compass, my search was aimless. I believed a diagnosis, a word scrawled across a prescription pad, would justify my experience. Instead, I had x-rays, MRIs, and scans "proving" my good health. Blood tests showed an elevated ANA (antinuclear antibody), and my titers tested positive for tick-related disease, yet no official diagnosis materialized.

Specialists gave isolated, conflicting opinions. I was tested for dozens of conditions including multiple sclerosis, lupus, arthritis, ankylosing spondylitis, stroke, and Lyme disease. My results showed indicators for Rocky Mountain spotted fever, lupus, rheumatoid arthritis, connective tissue disease, paresthesia, myasthenia gravis, and Reynaud's phenomenon. Yet, the diagnoses were inconclusive. I had parts of each of these illnesses but not the whole.

> "*An imaginary ailment is worse than a disease.*"
>
> —Yiddish Proverb

One cardiologist became angry at my frustration. He said, "You should be happy that there's nothing wrong with you! Do you want cardiomyopathy?"

Chastised yet again. His insult showed a gross lack of understanding. Of course I didn't *want* a heart condition. He failed to grasp the great chasm between "nothing wrong" and "we don't know what's wrong."

ℒ

The United States toppled a foreign dictatorship faster than I secured a diagnosis. Dr. Y returned from active duty, and I could barely wait. I was *finally* going to find out the name of my illness. I'd seen a flood of doctors, had a flood of tests. Previous doctor visits failed to provide answers, but this was different. My "real" doctor would give me the real scoop.

Sue's Symptoms List

- Life-altering widespread pain (joints, muscles, bones)
- Irritable bowel syndrome
- Balance/dizziness/coordination problems
- Overwhelming fatigue
- Painful tingling/burning/numbness (neuropathy) in extremities
- Headaches/migraines
- Insomnia and sleep problems
- Chronic bruising
- Squeezing chest pain/ heart palpitations
- GERD (gastroesophageal reflux disease)/acid reflux
- Thinning (disappearing) eyebrows
- Hair loss (bald spots)
- Skin discoloration (particularly across the face)
- Symptom flares
- Weight gain/abdominal swelling
- Yeast overgrowth
- Swallowing difficulties (a choking feeling)
- Chronic nausea
- Vision problems including an ocular migraine
- Malnourishment
- Difficulty gripping items
- Muscle twitching/shaking/tremors
- Heightened sensitivity to smells (cleaning chemicals, paints, fragrances, bug sprays, etc.)
- Fuzzy thinking/memory loss
- Female problems (PMS, fibroids)
- Nightly muscle cramps/spasms
- Inability to multi-task (sensory overload)
- Ringing in ears
- Fevers/chills/inability to regulate body temperature
- Severe carbohydrate cravings
- Chronic bronchial and respiratory infections / never-ending cough, to the point of vomiting
- Weak/impaired immune system
- Chronic toothaches and jaw pain

I slumped on the exam table; pain depleted all energy. My slate of symptoms had swollen in his absence. If Dr. Y listed all my symptoms in one place, it would have looked like the table to the left.

He glanced from my chart to me. Reacting to my dejected posture, he sounded annoyed. "You used to smile! You always told jokes. What's wrong with you?"

Wasn't *he* supposed to tell *me* that?

My brain felt fuzzy. Overwhelmed by disappointment, I had nothing to say. He fidgeted through my silence and looked back to my chart. His face suddenly brightened. "I think I have something."

The beginnings of hope surged.

"Your cholesterol is a bit elevated. There's a new med that'll fix you up in no time. I've got samples in my office."

There went the hope. I felt hollowed out, empty. I'd placed too much importance on this visit. I expected "the answer." I was wrong. Again.

Already taking more pharmaceuticals than a Jacqueline Susann character, I politely declined. If I'd had the clarity to speak (which I did not), I could have described for him how disappointed he made me feel by suggesting such a relatively trivial cause for what was by then *years* of misery.

Cholesterol wasn't my problem, and I knew it. Too tired for anger, I recognized that my faith in Dr. Y had reached an impasse. I had nowhere to turn. I needed those in the medical community to assign a diagnosis but no longer trusted them to find it.

As a Wiki Wiki bus driver once said in Hawaii, I was "between a hard rock and a fireplace."

ges

Solving my own health mysteries overwhelmed me. Too much responsibility. I was Dorothy looking for a yellow brick road — sans helpful companions. As a kid, I loved watching *The Wizard of Oz* on TV, but, I have to admit, I liked the commercials just as much.

Mattel, Hasbro, and Ideal ads were futuristic, modern. I coveted an Incredible Edibles machine to make Creepy Crawlers with root-beer-flavored Gobble-Degoop. In the midst of such Saturday morning commercials, one stood out like homespun muslin in a sea of lime-green polyester. In particular, a commercial for a memorization game called Hūsker Dū featured children dressed as if they shopped from missionary barrels. Fawning parents hovered over the too-polite kids. A goofy voiceover said, "Hūsker Dū! Do *you* remember?"

It was a simple game. Small pictures, visible through cutouts, were covered with markers. Players removed the markers two at a time, hoping for a match (Concentration-style). Improving my memory didn't impressed me, but it's claim to teach kids how to outwit their parents did. If I could outwit my parents, maybe I'd become good enough to beat my sisters?

Decades later, I played a grown-up version of Hūsker Dū on my dining room table. I arranged file folders, attempting to match symptoms with possible triggers. I sorted through medical receipts, test results, and print-outs from online medical diagnosis and treatment sources. The materials grew too cumbersome, and I realized a computer spreadsheet was necessary. Logging in the "knowns," I plotted symptoms, dates, and duration of illnesses, finally arriving at a big picture.

A pattern took shape. I saw periods of symptom flare-ups and noted commonalities. While stress remained a constant factor, I noticed other triggers. Odd occurrences, such as a course of antibiotics or a trip to the dentist, seemed to precede a flare. I searched online for a connection between my symptoms and a disease. I finally handwrote a list of possible illnesses and compared each condition to my symptoms. I matched them one by one, Hūsker Dū-style. Some conditions related to some of my symptoms, but only one showed a potential relationship to all of them.

I connected the dots and arrived at my own hypothesis: *fibromyalgia* — often considered a diagnosis of exclusion — a label affixed once every other possible consideration is ruled out.

> *If we put everything in the hands of experts and if we say that as intelligent outsiders we are not qualified to look over the shoulder of anybody, then we're in some kind of really weird world.*
>
> —Michael Chrichton

After a decade of wondering, including a total of three years of intensive search for a diagnosis, I'd *never once* had the term fibromyalgia suggested to me. Not from *any* health practitioner — professional or otherwise. During that time, I was consistently told I was fine after each medical test. No illness. No disease.

I visited a new doctor armed with backup data. I presented my three-page spreadsheet to Dr. Z, pointing to columns of information and dates and durations of symptoms. I pleaded my case. Saying the word "fibromyalgia" out loud for the first time felt devastating. To me, the word dangled in the air like a noose.

Dr. Z said, "No-duh."

She directed her next comment to the intern at her side. "This isn't normal. Patients don't usually have the research done and the answers ready for you."

She noted my official diagnosis on my patient chart.

Hmm … so this is what it feels like to "have the answer." Instead of sitting like a dishrag on the exam table, I felt empowered. I chose to participate in, rather than be a spectator of, my own health management team. In fact, I was the team captain.

Imagine that!

"Wisdom becomes knowledge when it is personal experience."

—Unknown

Chapter 3

Welcome to Fibroworld: You are here (X).

finally had a diagnosis: fibromyalgia. I belonged to a community of others with shared experiences. I learned that before I could move forward, I had to understand where I was. What was fibromyalgia, anyway?

ঞ

My first exposure to the word "fibromyalgia" was in the early nineties on a book cover featured in a Harriet Carter catalog. The adjacent product was a golfing toy designed to use "while on the potty." That didn't lend much credence to the subject matter.

After confirmation of my diagnosis, however, I became a (web) Surfing Pro. I wanted to know everything about this condition that seemingly defined my life. In the new millennium, only slightly more information existed online. I surfed through the meager treatment options and repeatedly found myself directed to Dr. Joseph Mercola's medical website.[1] Dr. Mercola's advice was simple (too simple, I thought). It seemed no matter what the illness, his suggestions were constant: a holistic diet and exercise. Terms such as *whole foods, organic, toxicity,* and *processed foods* swirled at me like insults. Gee, my diet wasn't that bad; was it?

Was I to have a life deprived of fare as American as apple pie? *Get real!*

However, I soon learned that simple does not mean simplistic. Sometimes fundamental truths *can* filter down to a few key principles.

ঞ

---

1. Dr. Joseph Mercola, http://www.mercola.com/ [accessed 02/02/10]

Let's face it: If fibromyalgia weren't such a pain, it'd be funny. It's the most infuriating "invisible" condition you'll ever not see. Medical sources differ on where to categorize it. I first learned it was considered an autoimmune disease. I studied the near one hundred conditions on the American Autoimmune Related Diseases Association website.[2] I reviewed each one and zeroed in on conditions with familiar symptoms: lupus, rheumatoid arthritis, multiple sclerosis, Guillain-Barre, Epstein-barr, chronic fatigue, mixed connective tissue, Reynaud's phenomenon, and Crohn's disease, among others. Many of us have a Heinz 57 version of chronic illness: a little bit of this and a little bit of that. I refer to my personal unofficial diagnosis as an "autoimmune cocktail."

Technically, fibromyalgia is not a disease but rather a syndrome, meaning no underlying etiology (cause) exists. Rheumatoid arthritis and multiple sclerosis also fit in this category. The word *syndrome* makes me think of the super-hero-wanna-be from the 2004 Pixar film, *The Incredibles*. He chose the name Syndrome so he could *be* somebody. His jet-black bodysuit featured a bold "S." His crowning glory — a cape. For now, syndrome is the term we fibrofolk "wear."

Fibromyalgia patients are no longer referred primarily to rheumatologists. Fibromyalgia has been reclassified from rheumatologic to neuralgic, from blood to brain. The world over, rheumatologists are heaving a sigh of relief, while neurologists are starting to bite their nails.

It makes sense that fibromyalgia is a brain-related condition (and *not*, technically, autoimmune). Stress is a primary fibromyalgia trigger. Stress begins in the brain, having both a mental and physical impact. The fight-or-flight phenomenon demonstrates how stress affects the body. Under duress, stress chemicals wash over portions of the brain that regulate pain sensitivity. When danger subsides, stress chemicals diminish. For fibrofolk, the brain gets "stuck" in stress mode.

Continuous bombardment of stress chemicals causes damage to the nerve control centers in the brain. Yes, that's brain damage.

The reclassification of fibromyalgia as a neurological condition made sense to me. Pieces of my diagnosis puzzle were beginning to make a clearer picture. I began to identify with my condition and feel a sense of belonging. However, that sense was more a matter of

---

2.   http://www.aarda.org/ The American Autoimmune Related Diseases Association [accessed 01/08/10]

resignation than acceptance.

A fibromyalgia diagnosis is like an invitation, Mafia-style, to a club you'd never otherwise frequent. An offer you can't refuse. Gnarly hazings and secret handshakes vary per club, but the commiseration over symptoms is universal. Extraneous symptoms differ, but these three dominate: pain, fatigue, and fog (cognitive difficulties). I call them the "Fibro Trifecta."

For a cohesive community feeling, I think a fibromyalgia diagnosis should come with a universal care packet. Similar to a "you are here" marker at the mall, it would give you a sense of your whereabouts. Included should be a fibromyalgia survival guide, a veggie-and-nut basket, a T-shirt emblazoned with a magenta "F" and, of course, a cape. It takes superhuman powers to get through each day with fibromyalgia, so why not wear a cape?

The most frustrating comment I (and others) hear is, "It's all in your head." Technically true, but an ignorant over-simplification of what those of us with the big "F" deal with on a daily basis. Feel free to borrow my retort: "Yes, fibromyalgia is in my head. That's where *my* brain is located. Where's *yours*?"

Maybe someday I'll even say it out loud.

৪৯

Documented cases of public figures dealing with fibromyalgia are pretty scarce. Considering it took until 1990 to formally establish diagnostic criteria, I have to give historians some slack.

Only a few celebrities have publicly disclosed their diagnoses, and why would they? Public scrutiny and potential un-insurability affects celebs and non-celebs alike. It takes courage to become aligned with such a misunderstood condition.

As a history buff, I've compiled a list of famous people who likely lived with fibromyalgia. Working backward through time, I've included a famed few who've tread this wobbly path before me.

Mexican-born artist Frida Khalo (1907-1954) suffered for her art. She suffered for her relationships. She just plain suffered. Her lifelong pain condition was most likely fibromyalgia, and it showed. Of her one hundred and forty-three paintings, fifty-five are self-portraits, the majority depicting her experience with pain. Unibrow not withstanding, most of us fibrofolk recognize ourselves in her work.

The 2002 Hollywood biopic brilliantly portrayed her misery … maybe too brilliantly. Merely witnessing Selma Hayek's artistic mood swings and angst was enough to send me into a symptoms flare.

Florence Nightingale (1820-1910) tirelessly cared for others, choosing squalor over the cushier surroundings of her upper-class birth status. Her body eventually gave out, and she became a world-famous invalid, bedridden for more than forty years. This earned her the title, "successful malingerer." Probably not a legacy she appreciated.

And now, the *pièce de résistance*: the most famous fibromyalgia celebrity in history. She demonstrated grace under less-than-ideal circumstances. Her sensitivity to pain identified her, but she used that skill to further her career. She wore her hyper-awareness with the dignity and grace befitting royalty. In fact, she was royalty.

Her story, as documented by beloved author Hans Christian Anderson, is one of obscurity, discovery, and fame. I'm referring, of course, to the *Princess and the Pea*.

> *"I didn't ask to be a princess, but if the crown fits..."*
> —Unknown

The tale begins with her knocking on a castle door late one rainy night, arriving bedraggled, befuddled, and bereft (definitely fibromyalgia). She declares herself a princess in need of a good night's sleep.

The dubious Queen Mum has a room readied, instructing servants to stack twenty mattresses and twenty eiderdown quilts over one measly dried pea.

The princess spends a sleepless night trying to avoid the hardened pea as it presses into her fragile body. Royal purple bruises bear proof. At breakfast, she complains of her terrible experience and haughtily blames the lumpy mattresses.

She is proclaimed a true-blue royal, and the queen bows to the delicate princess. The queen confesses her error in judgment and then utters my favorite line: "Nobody but a real princess could be as sensitive as that."

Analytically, the princess is lost, delusional, a hypochondriac. Yet, she's defined as *delicate*. Has a doctor ever said to you, "Aren't you a delicate thing?"

I hereby formally amend my declaration that a fibromyalgia diagnosis be accompanied by a cape: It should come with cape *and* crown!

ℱ☙

One morning I woke with my right wrist and forearm in terrible pain. They throbbed as if I'd played weekend tennis with a bowling ball. I was sure something was terribly wrong, and I searched through a junk drawer for my old wrist brace.

Because of the pain, I skipped the gym and headed straight home after work. I later sat at my computer and absentmindedly picked up a glob of rubber cement I'd peeled from a junk mail credit card offer the day before. I had rolled the two-karat-sized ball back and forth between my thumb and middle finger the prior afternoon as I worked. Zap! Pain shot through my hand and forearm as I repeated the move.

Unbelievable. I was actually wearing a wrist brace for a rubber-glue-ball injury.

Fibromyalgia pain is near impossible to anticipate. I blame it on "dain bramage." If my brain transmits a DEFCON TWO alert to my muscles for something ridiculous, how can I predict my pain level for something ordinary?

I once wrenched my back and shoulders from picking up a purse loaded with an extra book. I suffered a weeklong crick in my neck from tripping over a rug. A three-day heating-pad bender followed a day of wearing a new jacket with a heavy, faux-fur-lined hood.

Yes, these are true fibro-weird stories. That something so minor, so insignificant, can impact health defies logic or prediction. This is the reality for those of us with this diagnosis. Even our own reflections are incongruent with our feelings. We hear, "Gee, you look fine," but if we looked as bad as we sometimes feel, it would be Sasquatch returning our stare in the bathroom mirror as we brushed our teeth.

It's understandable why doctors can't figure it out. As patients, we test their patience. I wasn't surprised when I tripped over this tidbit of information online—a "diagnostic" mnemonic device used in jest (right?), but a glimmer of truth shines through. An anonymous doctor instructed his interns to look for four things when assigning a fibromyalgia diagnosis: Pain, Energy decrease, Sleep disturbance, and

Tender points. See the acronym? There you have it: P.E.S.T.

Fibromyalgia is confounding. It's no wonder that "normals" (as opposed to fibrofolk) don't know what to expect from us. We need to make it clear to friends, family, and coworkers that we don't expect them to anticipate our needs. How could we ask it of them when we're simply trying to stay one step ahead of it ourselves?

৪৯

Have you ever heard of odor layering? Dogs do it; people can't. A dog can discern individual odors rather than one all-encompassing enticing aroma.

> FIDO: Mmm ... a whiff of week-old Taco Bell, ratty running-shoe insoles, and beach towels moldy with San Clemente runoff water. Awesome!

> ME: My kid's closet smells like a fertilizer factory.

As odor layering is to smells, my personal archeology skills are to pain. I've learned to identify individual characteristics of my pain rather than feeling it as one entity. I can identify the type, onset, origin, and possible trigger — a skill honed from experience.

I've named my pain varieties: Lighthouse, Sandpaper, Taser, Joan Crawford, Dead Weight, and Puddling. There are headache varieties, too: Hat and Nickel.

Lighthouse pain happens in my joints and bones. It's a pulsing, low-grade throb followed by a sharp jab. The dull-dull-dull-*sharp* pattern reminds me of a revolving lighthouse beam.

Sandpaper pain happens in my joints, most commonly in the hips. The joints feel sandpaper-lined and grind when I walk. I notice it most when climbing stairs.

Taser pain happens in my chest. Rapid and knife-like, it feels like a micro-pointed electrocution. These episodes are short-lived, and, thankfully, I'm not.

Remember Joan Crawford's square-shouldered jackets? The pain sometimes feels as if two anvils are balancing like lead shoulder pads. The downward pressure is so intense, I wonder if it were somehow relieved, would I float to the ceiling?

Dead Weight pain is heavy, burning, and tingling in the muscles. I picture millions of microscopic Pacmen chomping through muscle fibers, causing them to leak tiny, pain-filled battalions into the area. These pain battalions multiply and spread, causing generalized tenderness, heaviness, and inflammation.

Dead Weight pain affects entire limbs or large areas of the body such as the back, neck, and shoulders. I suffered Dead Weight pain for several years in my left arm. Constant tingling and limited sensitivity in my fingers made it difficult to grip. A chronic case of the dropsies resulted in much shattered glassware.

> "*Pain is the root of knowledge.*"
>
> —Unknown

Dead Weight pain is affected by sleep. Sleeping well (reaching the stage of restorative benefits, REM stage) typically improves morning pain level. Yet, I've noted that morning pain *increases* after a night of deep sleep. While it seems contradictory, I believe it's a result of lack of circulation — less tossing and turning. Happily, though the pain is greater, it fades more quickly. After a night of poor sleep, the pain lingers for most of the morning if not the whole day.

I call the point of pain fade "burnoff," similar to the evaporation of the foggy marine layer in coastal areas. Everyone is different. The point where your morning pain recedes depends on overall health, fitness, stress levels, and sleep quality. For these reasons, I believe that burnoff is a better indicator of health than the actual pain level. (See further discussion in Chapter Six.)

Dead Weight pain is often accompanied by pain Puddling — an accumulation of increased pain in dense patches within the greater area of pain. Puddling collects pain similar to condensation trapped between two sheets of glass. And, like trapped moisture, you know it's there but can't do a thing about it.

My pain Puddling often centers near a former injury. If you've had surgery, a broken bone, or tissue damage, you may experience chronic pain Puddling in those areas.

My pain expertise has given me the ability to physically identify and differentiate among my muscles, organs, nerves, joints, bones, and even the vascular system.

Sometimes I get a feeling of constriction in my veins, as if they're seizing up and not allowing blood to flow properly. This can happen in my legs, but most often it's in my neck, chest, or upper left arm. I'm not sure how, but I believe blood flow constriction (ischemia) is linked to fibromyalgia.

My headaches fall into two categories. Hat headaches are all-encompassing. It feels as if a too-snug hat is smooshed onto my head, squeezing vise-like from all directions. A Hat headache can affect only the crown or the whole head, either a beret or a beanie. A Nickel headache is a singular spot of persistent pain (roughly the size of a nickel). A Nickel headache can occur anywhere on the head, and the intense throb can be quite alarming.

There you have it, my treatise on pain. Are you a pain expert, too? Admittedly, this hard-earned expertise comes from a field of study I didn't choose, but I accept the title of pain archeologist with grace.

ℒᗡ

After securing my official diagnosis, I had time to stew about Dr. Y's "cholesterol cop out." The more I thought about it, the angrier I became. I knew my elevated LDL levels were not the cause of my problems. Besides, they were hereditary not dietary!

I formulated a plan. I'd implement it and the "new and improved" me would march back to Dr. Y's office to show him how wrong he was. My plan wasn't rocket science; I'd eat right and exercise. I added more vegetables to my diet and stopped empty-calorie snacking. I exercised on my home treadmill after work and didn't eat at all after dinner. This was the extent of my strategy.

I noticed changes almost right away. The first thing to grab my attention was the absence of chest pain. The squeezing feeling in my chest had become so familiar I almost missed it. I'd experienced GERD, gastroesophageal reflux disorder, for years (especially in the evening). Strangely enough, the pain simply vanished. So did my swallowing difficulty. Were the improvements imagined? Within a few weeks, however, there was no question. My new lifestyle proved positively beneficial. Gee, diet and exercise. Who knew?

Encouraged, I kept at it. After about four months, *all* my symptoms had improved. At six months, only a few remained, and even they were significantly diminished. And the side effects of my new lifestyle? Besides feeling great, I dropped unwanted pounds — about fifteen percent of my bodyweight.

I forgot all about revisiting Dr. Y. I felt better than I had in decades. I regained health by taking personal responsibility for my actions. Did it matter that my success stemmed from an obstinate plan to prove a point? Nope.

Kudos to Norwegian stubbornness.

For the record, I later had my cholesterol rechecked, and I was right. My HDL/LDL numbers changed little. I do have hereditary "high" cholesterol. I was the picture of health, at my ideal weight, and more fit than as a teen. Of course, being right was moot since, in attempting to fix one small problem, I fixed nearly all of them.

My catalog of complaints was all but tamed (I was about eighty percent pain-free), but I wanted to know why I was so much better. I sought enlightenment from peers at a local support group. Many others had similar frustrations with the medical community. The leader shared her own hurtful experience with a less-than-helpful doctor. When first diagnosed, she appeared afraid. Her doctor snapped, "Oh, don't worry. You won't die from fibromyalgia, although you'll wish you would."

Heavens! That was supposed to be helpful?

Wait while I climb up on my soapbox for this: It's often said that fibromyalgia is not life-threatening. That is true. However, while it's not life-threatening, it is definitely life*style* threatening. That's something to think about.

Doctors are only able to dispense advice from the information they're given. Some have little education or experience with chronic illness. That's the nature of things. Illnesses *become* chronic because the underlying problems are left untreated.

Encouraged by my own success, I sought atypical treatments, ones off the beaten path. I needed balance. Searching, I looked between the information that I thought was true and new "truths" as they unfolded.

"The beginning of knowledge is the discovery of something we do not understand."

—Frank Herbert

Chapter 4

Lessons Learned While Navigating the Misinformation Superhighway

o, I got a grip on what gripped me — fibromyalgia. I'd learned how to keep it from getting worse, but could I make it better? And if so, how much? Creating an action plan, I searched for further answers, solutions and, for the first time in my adult life, balance.

Living with chronic illness is enlightening. After all, people trek to mountaintops simply to better understand themselves. This is true: You'll never know your body better than when it screams for attention every day. You may not want to listen, but you *have* to listen.

Listening is the key to wellness.

Listening is so vital it's more than the key. It's also the lock, the gate, and the drawbridge over the moat. Listen to your mind and body. Listen to the advice of others (take in the good stuff and dump the junk). Listen to your inner voice and pave a path toward healing. Seek solutions to your own personal health questions.

Being proactive means storming your own castle.

ॐ

Knowing what I have, at least, I laughed, I cried, and I spent a fortune on alternative medicines. My first experience with a complementary medical practitioner (other than a chiropractor) was before my diagnosis and beyond strange. It set the stage for the unusual and wonderful practitioners I'd yet to meet. Referred by several reliable sources, I'd heard different accounts of his methods. All agreed on his diagnostic acumen.

One friend called him Dr. Chickenbone, stating his methods

seemed akin to reading taro cards and tea leaves. Yet, he was one out of dozens of doctors to properly diagnose her son's elusive condition.

I half-expected a wizened, hunched guru in a hooded robe. Instead, I found a quirky, good-humored man fond of aloha shirts. He didn't take my medical history. He didn't take notes about previous diagnoses or current symptoms.

He also didn't take insurance.

Using Contact Reflex Analysis, also known as CRA® (a form of applied kinesiology), he immediately said a portion of my brain, the hippocampus, didn't work well. He used the word "damaged" and asked about head injuries. Next, he said my thyroid was almost non-functioning, but that concern was secondary. The hormonal imbalance causing my "female problems" was so pervasive, it needed immediate correction. And then there was the issue of my iodine deficiency.

I was disappointed. He missed my biggest concern: a constant and chronic squeezing pain in my chest/heart area (a symptom rudely dismissed at three separate cardiologist visits).

He summed up. "You've been seriously ill for a long time. You've stripped your gears, so to speak, and your adrenal and immune systems are shot. Your hormones are wacky, and your thyroid has given up. Clearly, you've been under a lot of stress, and it's put an overwhelming burden on your heart. Being so overworked, it probably hurts a lot."

Allrighty then … to whom do I write the check?

⅌⅏

It's important to know what type of students we are.

Let's say your car makes a funny noise. When the subtle whine becomes a definite rattle, do you:

    A) Pop open the hood and have a look-see?
    B) Drive it until the rattle (or the car) stops?
    C) Turn up the radio?

I admit to being a natural B (ignore the problem entirely), but I'm making efforts to override that inclination. I'm an A-in-training. I try to pay attention to little things before they become big things.

Several summers ago, I headed straight to my doctor after waking with a small bump on my cheek. I thought about ignoring it, but it was tender to the touch and felt hot. I expected the doctor to send me home with a pat on the head. I was sent home — *to lie down.* I also got a lecture about the serious nature of staph infections.

Knowing my reluctance for medications, my doctor placed her hands on my shoulders and said, "This is extremely important. You must take this antibiotic until it's gone. Doctor's orders."

Cs are rife with rationalizations. *I don't have the time or money for this. I don't know a good mechanic.* In the long run, excuses are never part of a good maintenance program.

Keeping the body running at optimum efficiency takes tinkering. Don't wait until your rattle has turned into a ker-thunk before doing something about it. I've learned a thing or two. Now, when I notice a knock in my motor, I pop the hood (so to speak) for that much needed look-see.

ஒ

Research and education have paved my personal path to wellness. As intrigued as I am with the abundance of information available online, there is also the potential for misinformation. I find reliable sources I trust.

I shouldn't have to say this, but blogs and chat rooms are not vetted medical sources. Neither are many "health-related" websites. That doesn't mean you won't find valid information, but it does mean you need to do the legwork to verify the facts. Blogs seem to act as a "watering hole" for fibro-newbies. That's not a bad thing; I wish I'd had that resource when I originally searched for information. It seems to me, though, that blogs and chat room threads belong to one of two categories: hopeless or hopeful. I follow the ones that dance to a merrier tune.

When something unverified piques my interest, I look for a corroborating source. Accurate information may not appear in exactly the same way from site to site, but the gist should be clear.

I read more medical journals and abstracts than I used to. Familiarity with terms and medical vocabulary is a natural byproduct of research. I'm usually able to pick out the key idea from the jargon.

I'm a bookworm. I digest what I read, draw my own conclusions, and don't disparage the source. One of the most important medical discoveries for me came years ago from a chat room discussion group on chronic pain. I desperately sought a name for the constant squeezing in my chest. Remember the agony I described after my kitchen table incident?

I noticed dialogue about how chest pain mimics heart attack. I read an unfamiliar term and wrote it on a scrap of paper: costochondritis. I searched for more information, finding little. I now know it's a painful condition marked by inflammation of the cartilage connecting the ribs to the breastbone. Pain levels vary from mild to excruciating and can last for many months.

I took a computer printout regarding costochondritis to Dr. Z, and she did some research on her own. Agreeing with the diagnosis, she made suggestions, including that I look into stress-relieving techniques. I finally had a name for my chest pain! Sometimes names *are* important.

Unearthing that nugget of information was a giant step forward for me. As with panning for gold, it takes patience and tenacity to find answers. The validation of my chest pain experience helped me heal.

↬

After a chronic illness diagnosis, "guaranteed to work" remedies seem to creep up everywhere. Snake oil and voodoo, some say.

I've found as many people who swear *by* a remedy as those who swear *at* it. To each his own. Results depend on the individual nutritional needs of the individual body. Yes, lives have been changed by "miracle" products, but there's usually a nutritional and emotional component to that healing. Rather than finding yourself swayed by the claims of a product, learn what's in it and what it can offer.

Sometimes, products considered miraculous in the past seem to stop working. Maybe the body's needs have changed. Search for alternatives, and read the labels of every product you consider. Be relentless in your pursuit of health.

Healing happens in phases. We try new things; some work, some don't. We have phases of improvement and times when it seems little or nothing is happening. At all times, listen to your body, learn from the experience, and keep going.

How do you know if a supplement is working? Clues can pop up in unexpected places. Signs such as reduced swelling or pain relief are obvious, but others might be more subtle such as ones reflected in your mirror.

Blotchy skin, thinning hair, brittle nails, and burning, dry, or bloodshot eyes can all be symptoms of illness. Changes in physical characteristics can herald improved inner health.

I've experienced many physical improvements that I attribute to vitamin supplementation. I add new supplements or products one at a time to give each a fair analysis. Most miracles don't happen overnight, so if I plan to spend the time and money on a product, I consider taking it for a reasonable length of time. It may take as much as four to six months to judge the success or failure of a product (following instructions, of course). Contrary to the advertisements, instant results are rare. Remember that it took years to create a chronic condition, and it takes time to turn health around.

> *"Never discourage anyone who continually makes progress, no matter how slow."*
>
> —Plato

There's an added benefit to learning the pros and cons of supplementation. We receive free, at no additional charge, the bonus gifts of patience, persistence, and self-awareness.

❧

How would you care for a plant that you wanted to blossom? Provide properly amended soil, ample light, and water. In other words, create an environment for your plant that includes everything it needs.

Think about "growing" a condition such as fibromyalgia. If you wanted the symptoms to blossom, you'd create the perfect environment, right?

First, you'd involve yourself in as many stressful situations as possible: family drama, work overload, negative internal dialogue. Next, you'd model your physical activities after a hibernating bear. You'd allow your muscles to slacken and compromise your skeletal structure. Finally, you'd deprive your body of nutrition. You'd consume sugars and processed foods, known to promote aging and inflammation. Create this environment, and your "plant" is guaranteed to "blossom" with pain, deterioration, and disease.

At some point we have to ask: Are our expectations for improved health in alignment with our actions?

What better crusade is there than the protection of our own natural habitat? It doesn't work to take a passive role in your health maintenance. Choose to participate. Become your own personal environmentalist!

ஜ

A fascinating study on heart disease revealed the answer to a long-held question of mine. If stress can create chronic illness, why does the evidence show up later (sometimes years) *after* the stress has been relieved?

The most stressful decade of my life was the mid-eighties to mid-nineties; yet, for the most part, I was symptom-free at that time.

A German study (unfortunately, done with canine subjects) showed how stress, intentionally inflicted on a dog's life, caused internal inflammation. The dog developed stress-induced heart disease. It physically adapted to the disease and thrived even through the stressful situations. The dog's body gave out *after* the stressor was removed, and it died of a heart attack.

The study concluded that the dog had an amazing capacity to adapt to stressful situations. He, however, couldn't emotionally "let go" of the stress — even when the stress no longer existed.

Humans, too, have a superior capacity for adapting and surviving. We exhibit unbelievable stamina through the toughest of times, but that stress eventually takes a toll.

There is a definite link between the timing of stress and disease. This helped me understand how I endured an era of extreme stress but physically fell apart when the good times rolled in.

Yet another piece of my health puzzle snapped firmly into place.

ஜ

I'm always talking about health. I reply to questions about nutrition, exercise, and pain management in person, via email, and by phone. At the gym, while shopping, and in line at Disneyland, the topic prevails.

Discussing health issues is a growing trend for the general population, too. It's even more popular for chronically ill people corralled in close quarters. I'm referring to the local support-group scene. Ralph Kramden and Fred Flintstone went down to a lodge looking for understanding; fibrofolk head to their local support group. Support groups can be a great place to share helpful hints and ideas for health management.

But sometimes I'm frustrated by what I call the *battle of ills*. Attendees get excited to commiserate, but sharing often leads to comparing.

"My pain is so bad I can't walk farther than my mailbox."

"Really? You can get all the way to your mailbox? Lucky you."

Giving or receiving compassion is fine, but when some try to top others' complaints, conversation becomes like a computer program stuck in an endless loop. Nothing to do but reboot.

Some simply want a friendly soul to listen. It's taken me a while, but I've learned that it's not wise to interject helpful hints to people who are not ready, willing, or interested in hearing them.

Each person has to make the pilgrimage toward improved health in his own way or in her own time. *Where* you are on your journey affects your interpretation of information more than anything else.

Now when I'm referred to someone in crisis, I ask, "How long have you been sick?" There's never a short answer, but it gets me to my next point. Lessons are ready to be learned when we're ready to hear them.

Here it is again: Listening is an essential part of healing.

THE BREAKFAST MENU OF ACCEPTANCE

I've found that dealing with and accepting any chronic condition takes a person through three distinct stages reminiscent of the Kübler-Ross stages of grief. This is my take on these stages:

1) WAFFLES – First, we waffle. We experience wide mood swings. Like Sally Field's Sybil, we mutter conflicting dialogue: "I am sick. *No, I'm not.* I feel great. *I'm going to die.* My doctor's full of crap. *I'm full of crap....*"

This stage can go on for years, depending on one's personal history of dealing with tragedy and any available support systems.

2) PANCAKES – Next, we're overwhelmed. We accept that we have a chronic condition. We'll live under this onerous black cloud for the rest of our lives. We'll never be able to dot, dot, dot, ever again.

This stage is so vast and bleak we can't imagine living happily ever after. Health is the unachievable Rhett Butler. We don't have the energy for drapery dressmaking, and we're so far from well we can't recognize that Tara is within our grasp.

3) OATMEAL – Finally, we're balanced. Like Goldilocks, we find the "just-right" way to deal with our illness. We weave our newly defined existence into our old life. We're not the same as we once were — we're new and improved!

The Oatmeal stage brings self-knowledge. Through personal assessment, we can conclude that we have Tara; we know how to work the land, and we bear the blisters to prove it.

We've learned what works — and what doesn't. We do our own research. We graciously accept news clippings, forwarded emails, and ripped-out magazine articles sent from well-meaning friends and acquaintances. We read them and assess their practicality; WE determine their validity. We're on our way to a healthier future, and it all begins with knowing where we fit within the Breakfast Menu of Acceptance.

ॐ

Recognizing what Breakfast stage we're in is an important assessment. If we're Waffling, we can't process new ideas about healing and wellness. Why should we? We're not even sick!

If we're Pancaked, we may listen to information, but we can't take it in or apply it. "Sick Person" is our new job title. There's room for little else in our world. A person in the Pancake stage may say, "…but that won't work for me because…" or "I would love to try that but…."

Pancaked people have big buts. Whenever I hear "but" followed by an excuse for inaction, I imagine a brick in one hand and a trowel in the other. Each "but" is another brick mortared into a wall of excuses.

> "*Acceptance is not submission; it is acknowledgment of the facts of a situation. Then deciding what you're going to do about it.*"
>
> —Kathleen Casey Theisen

There's no one-size-fits-all health solution, but success comes to those who tenaciously pursue results. We have to start somewhere.

Humans have a tendency to over-think things. Our logical side holds us back from taking action. Forrest Gump's friend Bubba did not suffer that fate. Examples of his one-track mind made us laugh (shrimp kebabs, shrimp Creole, shrimp gumbo....), but his drive and initiative made us think. He had that "git 'er done" attitude.

In the Oatmeal stage, people process information by applying a skill a friend of mine calls "sifting": the ability to take in information as it applies to ourselves and ignore what doesn't. Once we're able to sift information, our learning potential and progress proceed full steam ahead.

How do these stages affect a person's perception of their illness? Wafflers give their condition no merit. They don't acknowledge their physical impairments: illness denied. In the Pancaked stage, the pendulum has swung too far toward "Woe is me, I am sick." Consumed by their own thoughts, they're overwhelmed. Those in the Oatmeal stage find the "just right" balance of *dealing* but not *dwelling*. With a firm grasp on the reality of the condition, the Oatmeal-stage person is still able to fold in new thoughts and ideas.

Information processing is clearly different for those in the Oatmeal stage. They're focused more on getting better than on limitations. Once they understand — and, of course, accept — their condition, they can work toward this goal.

What we CHOOSE to focus on is what we WILL attain.

As with anything worthwhile, this takes a bit of study. Going through each stage of understanding moves us forward. We can't skip through the process, but we can minimize the time spent learning these necessary lessons by accepting that they're simply phases. This, too, shall pass.

To achieve Oatmeal Nirvana, we must become informed. Research your condition. Research options. Research treatment alternatives. Read everything possible about your condition, then read more — and/or select DVDs, view Internet video clips, and contact local and national support groups.

The medical community is advancing, and new theories are turning into new management tools and treatments. Each person is unique. What works for one may not work for another. It's our job to find out what works for each of us. If someone suggests "take a pill," however, run!

One of my chief frustrations with fibromyalgia is its unpredictability. I could feel like a caffeinated Jack Russell terrier one day and more like a tranquilized koala the next. In the Pancaked stage, I mourned the loss of an orderly life. My uncertain future lay ahead. How could I ever again set goals?

As usual, real life seeped through the cracks and took over. After all, you don't typically see wedding RSVP cards like this:

_____ will attend (if she feels up to it).

I had to make plans, right?

Little forays such as weddings led to bigger forays, such as chaperoning a junior high marching band trip. Set the pace and keep moving ahead. I look at it this way: what's worse — feeling unwell and staying home or feeling unwell and doing something enjoyable?

What breakfast food do you see when you look in the mirror? Recognize it for what it is. If it isn't oatmeal, find a new recipe!

TUNE OUT AND TUNE IN

This updated mantra for today's healthy lifestyle (whether you have chronic illness or no health challenges) is about tuning out distractions, nonsense, and meaningless demands, and tuning in to your personal goals.

Self-awareness, although often misconstrued as selfishness, is beneficial to you and to everyone around you. Tuning out distractions that keep you suspended in the past gives your focus a one hundred and eighty-degree turn. You're wholly available to participate and be present in your own life.

It takes practice to tune out what isn't important and to tune in to what is. Go back to that key word, *balance*. Emotional balance is a natural result of discoveries made on the way to self-awareness. Three health-related concepts constitute lifestyle balance.

To achieve the ultimate state of wellness that awaits us — that we all deserve — we must find balance in what I call the *restoration trio*: nutrition, exercise, and emotional wellness.

How we think transforms into how we feel. Our inner thoughts play a dominant role in our recovery and, therefore, can't be overlooked. Our "get well" equation takes all three components to add up, so let's move forward. Our healthy future is just steps away.

"We're living in a world today where lemonade is made from artificial flavors and furniture polish is made from real lemons."

—Alfred E. Newman

Chapter 5

Eating for Wellness:
You're just fueling yourself!

ho doesn't have a love-hate relationship with food? We crave the foods we shouldn't and avoid the ones we should. Dietary experts aren't much help. They use complicated lingo and give contradictory advice. However, looking at the information as a whole helps to focus, to spot commonalities. Some nutritional truths ring true no matter the source. As information becomes less fuzzy, nutrition awareness sharpens.

Doctors and health gurus agree that Americans need to eat more fresh vegetables. That's a great starting place.

Initially, I improved my diet, hoping to drop a few pounds (and to disprove Dr. Y's cholesterol theory). My results exceeded my wildest expectations. My pain levels dropped along with the weight. The more veggies I ate, the more I craved. Crisp, fresh cucumbers, snow peas, broccoli, spinach, and green beans tasted *good* to me. Before, I thought salads were for bunnies. I began to think of them as meals. I added goodies such as nuts, beans, veggies, and fruits. My salads hopped from the briar patch to the dinner table.

Shocking bonus: The more good stuff I ate, the fewer cravings I had for the bad stuff.

Prior to taking charge of my health, I was nutritionally illiterate. As I re-evaluated what I thought I knew about nutrition, I discovered the destructive role my misperceptions played in my health. Once I'd kick-started my healthy eating program, I knew this for sure: the better I ate, the better I felt. Eating nutrient-dense, healthy foods reduced my dizziness, pain, and fatigue. I was onto something.

Discovering that I could eat my way to improved health, I became an enthusiastic convert. How revolutionary. I felt like Helen Keller at the water pump. I thirsted for nutritional knowledge.

Blueberries have anti-aging properties? Turmeric and cinnamon can reduce joint pain, while also helping to prevent cancer, heart disease, and Alzheimer's disease? Sign me up!

I scribbled lists of foods and their nutritive benefits. I did online searches of nutritional studies related to arthritis, cancers, and irritable bowel conditions. I checked out books from the library, watched PBS documentaries, and scanned medical journals, findings, and abstracts.

I plucked out kernels of applicable information. I learned what happens when broccoli and cinnamon go to war in a Petri dish with cancer cells (hint: cancer sends up a white flag). I digested (sorry) hundreds of "The Top Ten Foods That…." articles.

My husband mumbled "uh-huh" every time I discovered a "new" tidbit of nutritional news. Ironically, a decade prior, the health battle was his. Seven months after our first date, my then-boyfriend was diagnosed with Hodgkin's lymphoma. Like little else, chemo speeds up the "getting to know you" phase of a relationship. I say we dated in dog years.

> "*Let food be thy medicine, thy medicine shall be thy food.*"
> —Hippocrates

I wish I'd had a lick of health I.Q. back then. Nutrition is the perfect partner to medical science, particularly for cancer treatment. I'm certain now that jumping onto the holistic diet bandwagon would have sped up his recovery with added, far-reaching benefits. Instead, the subject was never discussed. Isn't that appalling? Nutrition wasn't addressed by a single doctor, nurse, phlebotomist, receptionist, or parking lot attendant.

My health crisis caused me to self-educate. Changing my dietary habits began a healthier future for me and for my family.

Helen Keller's future changed when her teacher, Annie Sullivan, helped her discover a world of words. Fibromyalgia is my Annie Sullivan, showing me a world of healing. For that, I'm thankful. Can you think of any "Annies" in your life? Grasp the message like Helen did — with both hands.

೪ು

Nutritional news is everywhere. Foodie articles link eating your way to a healthier future with powerhouse foods such as spinach, kale, cilantro, broccoli, and tea. What do they have in common? Color!

My early nutritional education reflects a curious relationship to all things green.

I grew up in the heartland of America: Iowa — land of fresh air and fresher food. Ironically, our "produce" came from tin cans with a Shrek-colored giant on the label. The only green veggie to grace my plate was an occasional pea in my creamed tuna on toast. I tucked them under my castoff crusts, letting my cat lick fingers under the table.

For those who have not had the pleasure, creamed tuna on toast is an unsophisticated marriage of flour, margarine, milk, canned peas, and canned tuna. Heat and pour generously over toasted white bread. (The dish resembles *Titanic's* disaster scene: a floating "plank" surrounded by flotsam peas and jetsam tuna.)

In my childhood, the dish was accompanied by this proverb of the poor Swedish housewife:

> *To market, to market to buy a pig roast.*
> *Home again, home again, Tuna on Toast.*

In my early teens, further education came from sharking church potlucks. I was a pastor's kid in a town of fewer than two hundred people. Where else would I go? Potluck dinners reigned supreme over the social events they followed. Hot and cold food tables were judiciously separated by a sea of folding chairs. Dessert tables lined up nearest the watchful eyes of the kitchen ladies.

Salads were sugary, never leafy. Lime-green Jell-O hid under pastel mini-marshmallow crazy quilts. Pudding and Jell-O salads were almost sacramental — canned fruit cocktail or pears optional.

Nosing around the church kitchen, I snitched sugar cubes hidden behind the moss-green boxes of altar candles. At youth group meetings, I swilled Yahoo Mountain Dew from algae-green bottles, the perfect chaser for gooey Rice Krispie treats tinted kelly green for St. Patrick's Day.

Lunches at my grandparents' farm formally rounded out my

dietary instruction. Light Karo Syrup sandwiches (white bread, margarine, and transparent corn sugar) were served on green milk glass plates at the kids' table. Each bite offered icy bursts of syrup across the roof of my mouth — the cold I suspect now a likely result of rapid disintegration of tooth enamel.

That Iowa farm yielded a kid-perfect combo: cornfields on the outside and corn syrup on the inside. It's funny how my affiliations with the color green later matured. Yes, my farm life experience was green, but, ironically, so was my nutritional acumen.

୨ର

I went from knowing nothing about nutrition as a kid to thinking I knew everything by my early thirties. I knew what foods "agreed" with me and which did not. Irritable bowel syndrome (IBS) is an indiscriminant educator.

Fresh fruits and vegetables were my Public (Restroom) Enemy Number One. The contents of my intestines liquefied with a simple serving of watermelon, apples, or carrots. I told a doctor I couldn't digest raw fruits or veggies. He shrugged and said, "Then don't eat them."

My thought process was accurate, but my hypothesis was faulty. "Real" foods didn't agree with me, but my conclusion as to why was wrong. I didn't understand the internal conflict between artificial (fake) and real foods. I didn't grasp the mechanics of digestion and what effect processed foods had on my intestines. My doctors didn't get it either.

In blaming fresh fruits and veggies for my digestive problems, I shot the nutritional messenger. I had a lot to learn.

RIVER OF LIFE

Most survivalists know the Rule of Three: Humans cannot survive more than three weeks without food, three days without water, or three minutes without air. Obviously, water is fundamental to all living things.

As adults, our bodies are made up of sixty to seventy percent water. It's important to keep our "tanks" filled to capacity. Adequate consumption is vital for digestion, regulating body temperature, joint tissue support, circulation, toxin elimination, even skin rejuvenation.

Rivers provide a great metaphor for the importance of water in our bodies. Rivers are a natural form of transportation, efficiently conveying passenger boats and cargo. They're symbolic of life, renewal, energy. Water flows through the body like a river. As a transportation system, it carries all elements exactly where they need to go. Here's a visual image for you. Imagine the water you drink as an internal river and the nutrients transported by it are like little rubber ducks. With plenty of water, the duckies happily bob their way in a line toward their destination. Yes, your ducks are in a row.

What happens if the volume of your river is reduced, say, cut in half? Your duckies slow down. Some get stuck, drifting to where there's little or no water flow.

What happens if your internal river is reduced to a trickle?

A digestive system made sluggish by dehydration is not pretty. Expecting your lunchtime hoagie to make its way through your digestive tract without water is like taking the wheels off your roller skates and still expecting to glide.

How much water should we drink? A likely answer is, probably more than we currently do. Many people don't know they're dehydrated. The fact that thirst often masquerades as hunger complicates matters.

Authorities differ on the exact amount of water we need, but this method from Dr. Batmanghelidj[3] is simple. Divide your current weight by two and convert to ounces. That's how many ounces you should drink daily — no complicated math. As an example, a one hundred and fifty pound person should drink approximately seventy-five ounces of water per day. You'll know you're getting enough water if the color of your urine is a pale yellow, the color of straw (keep in mind that some B vitamins, veggies, and supplements can alter urine color). NOTE: You may need to drink more water than this equation demonstrates if you are more physically active.

Drinking water becomes a habit once you make it a priority. Always keep water handy. Set a daily goal and track your progress.

---

3 Fereydoon Batmanghelidj, M.D., author of *Your Body's Many Cries for Water*

Drink from a measured container to make monitoring your progress easy. Go easy when increasing your intake. If you're a new convert (switching to water from sweet-tasting drinks), your tastebuds may find water to be lacking in pizzazz. Most flavored waters contain undesirable ingredients and should be avoided. However, I know of one brand that contains nothing artificial (although I'm sure there are others). Metromint® water[4] comes in a variety of minty/fruity flavors and can be consumed as is or diluted with pure water for a "hint of mint" taste. The more water you drink, the more you'll crave. And, the better it will taste to you.

Initially, you may notice increased trips to the restroom, but this should be a temporary inconvenience. The body regulates to the amount of water you're drinking, and the frequency of bathroom breaks should normalize. If nighttime trips to the bathroom are a problem, it's a good idea to limit water intake after the evening meal.

Of course, the source of water and the container you drink from are important, too. Avoiding tap water is a good idea. Many brands of bottled waters are simply tap water with an expensive (and landfill-clogging) bottle. Besides the environmental nuisance, the plastic can leach harmful chemicals into the water. It's best to drink your water from glass, stainless steel, or specially made plastic containers. Filtration equipment varies greatly from do-it-yourself pitchers to equipment that requires professional installation. Purchase the highest quality filtration system that fits within your budget. If you choose reverse osmosis filtration, be sure to add trace minerals *back into* the water, as filtration removes all minerals and heavy metals. Trace minerals can be purchased in drop form for easy application to drinking water.

For many people, an acidic imbalance in the intestines is the cause of yeast overgrowth (discussed in detail later in this chapter). You might consider drinking alkaline water[5] to help deal with this imbalance. You can test for this imbalance with pH test strips available at most drug stores or, better yet, from a nutritionist. Alkaline water can be used both to detoxify and as a preventive measure. If you live in Japan or Canada, the filtering equipment

---

4   http://www.metromint.com/ [accessed 01/31/10]

5   http://www.nubalance.com/ [accessed 01/30/10]

used to create alkaline or ionized water is considered a medical appliance and may be covered under some insurance plans.

Water is the essence of life. Adequate hydration helps body tissues as well as digestion. When the body is adequately hydrated, it shows.

≈

Comparisons of the standard American diet (appropriately, S.A.D.) and the European diet are often in the news. Why do Italians, for example, eat breads and pastas yet escape the obesity pandemic striking Americans?

That's an apples to oranges comparison. Differences exist in the specific ingredients used and in the harvest-to-table time frame. Another factor is that Italians can turn food preparation and dining into a three-act play. Eating slowly for the sheer pleasure of it is foreign to us "chow-down" Americans.

The ingredients in American bread, pastas, and snack items differ from that in countries around the world. Our out-of-a-box macaroni is not their made-from-scratch fettuccine. Our overly processed ingredients are nowhere close to "natural."

Look at the time span between harvest and the meal on your plate. It could be weeks, months, or even years. Fresh, as it applies to processed American foods, is not fresh elsewhere. Processed flour and sugar are almost eternally "fresh," affected by neither temperature nor time. Food manufacturers have engineered shelf-stable products that are quick to prepare. Speed and efficiency — the American way!

Of the many positive attributes assigned to Americans, resourcefulness is near the top. We preserve and package ingredients to make them convenient. The irony is, by extending our food's shelf-life, we compromise our own.

Most products on today's grocery store shelves have been so denuded of their original essential vitamins and minerals that they're unrecognizable to our digestive systems. Sadly, many people don't know what natural foods taste or look like.

At a fibromyalgia support group, I met Saki, who wanted relief from her joint pain. When asked about her diet, she responded,

"I only eat whole foods. No junk. I eat bread, cereal, and pasta." Insistent about her healthy diet, she went on to say that she only ate homemade casseroles, cookies, and cakes. That's healthy, right?

Saki's use of the phrase "whole foods" illustrated her lack of understanding. She mistook *processed* (and, therefore, NOT whole) ingredients for foods in their natural, original state.

Read a cereal box label. Whole grains have been ground and refined (eliminating the nutritious, germinated portion of the grain), bleached, dyed, and combined with a host of artificial additives. A processed product is guaranteed to provide what we expect: flavor, crunch, creaminess. We expect consistent taste and texture in our processed foods. No soggy cereals. No stale crackers. Our expectations are high.

Today's packaged foods are engineered for the perfect balance of taste and "mouthfeel." Didn't know there was such a thing? Mouthfeel defined: "the tactile sensation a food gives to the mouth."[6]

Think of common foods that feel creamy: ice cream, fancy whipped coffees, cheeses, dips, spreads, salad dressings, cookie fillings, etc. Though these foods *feel* creamy, they may or may not contain cream. They may not be dairy-related at all.

Along with mouthfeel, there's the expectation of volume or portion size. Would you feel cheated if a grande muffin were regular-sized? We ask food manufacturers to lower their products' calorie content, but how can they do that? Either they reduce portion size or scientifically/chemically alter the ingredients. The latter scenario is the genesis of "frankenfoods" — artificially engineered foods altered by genetics or chemicals.

So, are food designers and manufacturers to blame? Haven't they simply created the products we've demanded? Change follows direction from us, the consumers. It's our responsibility to let them know what we want.

We *say* we want healthier foods, but what do we purchase? When we demand healthier, fresher alternatives, they'll show up in greater varieties and, eventually, at better prices.

Prices are just beginning to drop for organic and specialty foods. That shift is a good sign of things to come.

---

6   http://dictionary.reference.com/browse/mouthfeel/ [accessed 01/27/10]

It's important to re-educate our minds AND our palates. We have to first change our expectations of how food should look, feel, and taste. After that, making healthier food choices becomes easier.

" Of we're not willing to settle for junk living, we certainly shouldn't settle for junk food. "

—Sally Edwards

❧

Here's my nutritionist's explanation of how digestion works, summarized in my own words (a simplistic overview, so any errors or omissions are solely mine).

The digestive system is like a big puzzle, every piece fitting together, forming a perfect picture. When we eat whole foods, the digestive enzymes recognize the corresponding food particles, and the puzzle pieces snap together. When we consume foods that aren't recognizable, the pieces don't fit. How these "unrecognized" foods are digested and eliminated depends on the health of the digestive tract. In an unhealthy digestive system, undigested food coats the walls of the intestines like the insides of grungy basement plumbing.

Years of eating processed foods and frequent antibiotic use took a devastating toll on my health. Because my body lacked the ability to eliminate "fake-food residue" from my digestive tract, I couldn't properly digest *any* food, not even healthy food.

Intestines are lined with tiny hairs called villi (think of an inside-out fuzzy caterpillar). The villus increases nutrient absorption and keeps food moving. When they are gummed up or inflamed, they can go on strike and lie flat against the intestinal walls. Lazy villi can become inactive, causing constipation. Conversely, when intestinal health is impaired, villi can become overactive (read: stimulus maximus). The effects of over-stimulated villi need no description.

This is an oversimplification of the digestion process, but I include it for two reasons. First, I want to provide a better background of my impaired condition mentioned in Chapter Two. My critical illness led to questions that doctors (unfamiliar with nutrition) couldn't answer. I don't wish that frustration on anyone.

It now makes sense. I was swollen *and* starving: malnourished. Only a healthy change in my diet led to the healing my body desperately craved.

If this is the beginning of your healing journey, understanding where you are today helps point you in the direction of where you need to go tomorrow.

Second, no matter what the state of your health, I encourage you to remove highly-processed foods from your diet. Start with removing trans fats and high fructose corn syrups (HFCS). I mean it. Right now. Go to your kitchen and start tossing. See that "diet" salad dressing with HFCS on the nutrition label? Throw it out. The fake cream cheese with partially hydrogenated oils? Give it the heave-ho. You have my permission!

GUT I.Q.

The simple act of eating causes a dietary chain reaction. Food digestion creates an insulin response affecting the metabolism. Eating foods that increase the insulin response slows the metabolism. When insulin levels are elevated by sugars and simple carbohydrates, the body wants to store the excess carbohydrates as fat.[7] When simple carbohydrates are *increased* the metabolism of foods is *decreased*. Because proteins are slower to digest than carbohydrates, they cause a slower-paced insulin response.

Carbohydrates are not universally "bad." In fact, a meal comprised of a majority of fiber-rich carbohydrates is ideal. Vegetables are fiber-rich carbohydrates and provide nutrients essential to rebuilding healthy digestion. Comprehensive information on how the metabolism works (and how to repair it) can be found in Dr. Mark Hyman's book *UltraMetabolism*.

When we eat, the body sets digestive enzymes into action. They work efficiently throughout the meal and for sometime afterward. Proteins and fiber digest at a slow, steady pace, satisfying hunger (satiety). Sugary foods, especially between meals, impair the pace of digestion. We feel hungry more quickly after eating sugary foods and are more likely to overeat as a result.

---

7   Dr. Joseph Mercola article, *The 10 Things That Will Cause You to Be Fat* http://www.mercola.com/ [accessed 02/02/10]

By combining both proteins and fiber-rich carbohydrates, we get the best of both worlds. Together, they provide the digestive system with a steady release of insulin and keep the metabolism operating at peak efficiency. As with the fabled tortoise and the hare, steady wins the race.

It's fine to eat healthy snacks (nuts, seeds, fiber-rich raw veggies), but nibbling on empty calories throughout the day throws your metabolism into the cellar. Sugary foods lead to insulin spikes followed by the predictable "crash and burn" feeling.

Are you familiar with the glycemic index? What about glycemic load? The glycemic index (GI) ranks carbohydrates by their effect on blood glucose (blood sugar) levels. Typically, blood sugar elevates two to three hours after consuming carbohydrates. Foods higher in sugar content, such as highly processed foods (breads, pastas, cereals, snack foods, etc.) have a higher GI rating than fiber-rich vegetables and some whole grains. Higher GI foods release glucose rapidly and can cause blood sugar spikes, which may promote disease. Lower GI foods release glucose into the bloodstream at a slower and steadier pace. Understanding the GI is particularly helpful for diabetics to maintain a consistent blood sugar level.

The glycemic load (GL) cranks the glycemic index up a notch and adds portion size to the equation. It rates foods based on glycemic index *plus* volume, providing a precise measurement of the effect a food has on the digestive system.

Understanding the GI and GL tables is important. Higher indexed foods are often linked with inflammation, leading to joint and muscle pain. Knowledge is power. Know where your favorite foods rank on the GI and GL tables. Decide which to limit or eliminate from your diet.

Many indexes can be found online and in various nutritional books. Dr. Phil McGraw's book *The Ultimate Weight Solution Food Guide*, is a statistical food manual broken down into easy-to-understand categories. Arm yourself with nutritional know-how.

Monitoring calories alone isn't enough. Along with GI and GL rankings, consider also metabolic or nutritional typing (customizing your diet to include foods beneficial to *your* particular metabolism). Dr. Joseph Mercola's book *Total Health Program*, is the leading guide on how to tailor a diet to your specific needs.

Do your own research and come up with the programs and combinations of methods that work best for you. I read of a dieter who, instead of giving up white bread, chose to pair it with prunes when he had a craving. Strange, but interesting. High-glycemic white bread eaten with low-glycemic prunes made a winning combo for him. What might work for you?

Eating lonely carbs (simple carbohydrates eaten alone) can be disastrous to blood sugar levels. Instead, pair mealtime carbs with healthy fats or proteins to mitigate sugar spikes.

No discussion on digestion and metabolism is complete without a nod to the premier nutrient, fiber. It's a carbohydrate the body does not digest. That's not bad; that's good for digestion. Fiber's not hard to find. A diet rich in vegetables and whole fruits (not juice) ensures a diet rich in fiber.

Understanding the importance of digestion is key. Did you know there are more neurotransmitters in your gut than in your brain?[8] So, pay attention the next time you have a "gut feeling" about something. Fine-tuning your diet provides benefits beyond your imagination.

The brain overthinks, but the gut tells it like it is.

※

These three words can change your life: Read nutrition labels. Even better, increase your label-reading I.Q. by reading between the lines. Terms like "all natural" and "natural flavorings" are ambiguous. In advertising-speak, they're "weasel words." They sound important, but don't actually mean much. Dig deeper. Read all the ingredients and if you're unsure, either don't buy the product, or contact the manufacturer. We have a right to know what's in the food we buy.

Products may feature bold promises across the package, but for the true story read the nutritional information label on the side, back, or bottom. Food manufacturers go to great lengths to disguise what they don't want us to notice. Like the great Wizard

---

8   Dr. Hyman's article *7 Keys to UltraWellness, Lesson 4* http://www.drhyman.com/ [accessed 02/02/10]

working in his Emerald City palace, some prefer to keep their business behind a curtain. Trans fat labeling is a good example of this deceptive practice.

Manufacturers are now mandated to label food items containing more than 0.5 grams of trans fats per serving. When this change occurred, some food manufacturers simply changed the serving size of products. When has anyone opened a box of itty-bitty cookies and had two? Just because the label states "no trans fat" does not make it so. Look for clues such as partially hydrogenated oils in the ingredients list.

Ever read the nutrition labels of fat-free foods? Some fat-free dressing labels read like a recipe for chemical stew. We'd be better off using a healthy oil and real lemon juice.

Yes, deciphering nutrition labels can be confusing. First of all, ingredients are listed by chemical compound and/or Latin names. Look up unfamiliar ingredients. Not all scary-sounding ingredients are bad. Become familiar with food additives. Additive lists (and definitions) are conveniently available online, as they are often too lengthy to print.

Next, familiarize yourself with serving sizes and portions. I recently spotted an absurd health claim on a box of sugary kid's cereal. It claimed to have less sugar than a popular adult cereal. I grabbed both boxes to compare. As suspected, the sugar-coated cereal suggested a tiny serving size. Ounce for ounce, it had a much higher sugar content, but you'd never know it if you didn't read and compare the labels.

A packaged fruit-and-nut mix showed a mere ninety-four calories per serving. Nuts and dried fruits are not low-calorie foods. Checking the label, it suggested a serving that amounted to approximately four almonds and six cranberries. Is that a sampling or serving? In either case, it's wholly unrealistic.

Consumer awareness (through educated label-reading) paves the way to healthier eating. But, we can't have everything. Replacing partially hydrogenated oils (PHOs) with healthier alternatives may increase calorie count or saturated fat levels, among other things. It's give and take.

Once educated, our purchases speak loudly. We don't govern what manufacturers put in their products, but we can be selective about what we buy. Be proactive. Make the best choices for you and your family. When it affects their bottom line (profit), food manufacturers will respond to our demands for healthier food choices.

Food labels are not always accurate, but it's a good place to start. Research before you shop. Use a search engine to locate websites with nutritional labeling information. When weighing nutritional advice, always consider the source. Case in point: Follow the United States Department of Agriculture's food pyramid — only if pyramid is your desired body shape. A diet comprised mainly of grains and dairy is beneficial to the agricultural industry, not to most people. It makes me wonder. What if nutritional guidelines were developed by the U.S. Fish and Wildlife Service instead? Maybe pheasant and trout would become nutritional requirements.

For me, knowing what's *in* food tells me *if* it's food. I no longer consider pre-packaged snack items food at all. Looking at the ingredients list, would I eat BHT or BHA alone? What about a spoonful of yummy benzoic acid? Just because the additives are mixed with copious amounts of salt, sugar, and fats, does not make them food.

Informed label-reading helps you make better food choices. Like a wellness barometer, reading more labels indicates fair nutritional weather ahead. Of course, best of all is buying foods with no nutrition labels: fresh produce.

୫ର

Nutrigenomics (or nutrigenetics) refers to the relationship between nutrition and genetics. In a broader sense, it may also refer to individualized pharmaceutical treatments. This exciting topic brings good news to those with chronic illnesses. Pairing treatments with a patient's genetic blueprint means specialized and focused healing.

Why does one food dramatically reduce inflammation in one person yet show marginal results for another? What supplements or pharmaceuticals work specifically for you, and at what doses? Combining treatments and genetics creates a tailor-made wellness plan.

This concept doesn't fit neatly into our one-pill-fits-all society. During my husband's chemo treatments, they delayed his regimen when his vitality plummeted. Others at the hospital fared better — especially women and children. When he brought it up, a physician's assistant said, "We don't have dosages for chemo down to a science yet. We go by weight, and big guys like you probably get more than you need. It may be overkill, but we have to follow established protocol."

Overkill? That's not a word anyone going through chemo treatment wants to hear. Who wants to be a medical guinea pig?

Nutrigenomics makes sense. Each person's makeup differs. We each process and metabolize things differently. I experienced this phenomenon for the first time in high school. I suffered side effects from a pain medication prescribed following a school bus accident. Reading the prescription label, the school nurse said that I *should* feel sleepy, groggy. Instead, I had a bad case of the jitters, shaking too much to write. She flipped through the *Physician's Desk Reference* and confirmed what she already knew. I snuck a peek at the book while she phoned my doctor. In small print I read: "can cause excitability in children."

When I pointed to the book, she rolled her eyes and said, "You're not a child." At fifteen I didn't think so, either, but my weight was far below average. The dosage was wrong.

Nutrition as medicine is nothing new, but it *is* cutting edge in the health-maintenance field. The term "nutraceuticals" refers to using extracts of plants and foods medicinally. Nutraceuticals can help prevent and treat chronic illness.

The alchemy of supplements is one of the most difficult concepts to explain. Supplements can be helpful, even necessary, to heal from chronic illness. Finding the right balance takes detective work. A professional holistic nutritionist can help find what supplement(s) work for you. I recommend keeping an open mind to new ideas and treatments.

A nutritionist, naturopath, or a functional medicine physician can test for nutritional deficiencies. Supplementation can repair broken body functions such as inflamed tissues and poor digestion.

Get energized about finding answers to your nutritional health questions. The restoration of your health is the reward.

&

Earlier I mentioned that I believed Dr. Mercola's nutritional advice was unrealistic. I decided that he was a kook because his remedy for nearly every disease distilled down to diet and exercise. For me, that "unrealistic" concept took time to sink in.

Simplicity can be deceptively complex.

Dr. Mercola's rise from kook to genius, in my mind, was a slow ascent. I struggled with his restrictive nutritional ideas, but his healing successes intrigued me. Many of his patients listed symptoms all too familiar. He shed light on the inconsistencies of western medicine and taught me how the pharmaceutical tail wags the medical community's dog.

Once these general concepts took root in my mind, nutritional empowerment was within my reach. Trading artificial foods for natural foods gave me a satisfaction both physical and emotional.

Empowerment took me by surprise at a local restaurant.

I love soup: an entire meal's worth of nutrition in one tidy bowl. I love the flavors of fresh, wholesome ingredients.

One day I ordered a bowl of chicken tortilla soup (sans tortillas) at a restaurant I hadn't been to in a long while. The soup's murky appearance surprised me. My first spoonful tasted like a glump of salty plastic followed by a metallic twang. Dripping from my spoon, it resembled motor oil from a dipstick.

> "*There ain't a body, be it mouse or man, that ain't made better by a little soup.*"
>
> —Cook from *The Tale of Despereaux* by Kate DeCamillo

I dissected bits of carrots and chicken from the broth, trying to discern individual flavors. Nope. The bowl was one cohesive swirl of "fake."

I couldn't wait to get home to brush my teeth — and my tongue.

The restaurant's recipe hadn't changed, but I had. Healthy eating had given my taste buds CPR, and they enjoyed every bit of the flavorful experience. I learned that my homemade "thin but zesty" soup overrules "thick and artificial" soup any day.

Mercola — a name right on the tip of my tongue.

✿

The word "nutrition" is an integral part of my health lexicon; I prefer it to the negative-sounding term "diet." Nutrition suggests *including* foods while diet focuses on *removing* food choices. Nutrition is an active, take-charge word.

Nutrition teaches us what foods fuel the body and what ones deplete our resources. In simple terms, I categorize foods into two groups: Green Light or Red Light.

GO! Green

When we eat, we refuel. The body converts food into energy to perform. It's consumed, digested, eliminated. Green Light foods provide abundant nutrition and digest efficiently. They include vegetables, fruits, whole grains, and lean proteins. Green Light foods are fairly simple to identify: They spoil.

Green Light foods work *with* your digestive system and then get the heck out of Dodge. Isn't that the goal? Ideally, the body extracts nutrients from foods, leaving digestive enzymes to break down and eliminate what's left.

Think about a freshly sliced apple on a plate. How long until it turns brown? The apple begins to biodegrade and spoil almost immediately. Foods that naturally decompose are generally easier to digest. Green Light foods are natural, whole, unprocessed.

Nuts and beans are Green Light foods, too, although they digest more slowly than vegetables or fruits. With Green Light foods, nutrition is primary, efficiency secondary.

Healthy eating means Going Green. Shop at nearby farmers' markets and purchase locally grown vegetables and fruits. Purchasing local produce reduces global fuel costs and emissions. Eating "green" also helps your body work at peak efficiency (reducing "personal" gas emissions, too). That's a good thing!

STOP! Red

Red Light foods take a more circuitous route through the digestive tract. They're often lower in nutritional value than Green Light foods and don't digest as efficiently. They include prepackaged foods, simple refined carbohydrates, and chemically altered cuisine.

This is an unsophisticated definition, but the distinction is important. Foods that do not eliminate efficiently may stick around. Over time, this can create a plethora of health problems. Food can begin to rot in the colon. Diverticulitis, a pit or bulge in the intestine, can result. Those areas can become inflamed, causing diverticulosis. These conditions are sometimes called leaky gut syndrome. It's obvious that food elimination is crucial to good digestive health.

Red Light foods can be tricky to identify. Enriched white rice is a Red Light food, while a true whole grain rice is not. (HINT: When you see "enriched" on the package, think "highly processed.") Consider the origin of a food. The further a food is from its natural state, the more likely it's a Red Light food. Overprocessing limits the nutritive value of Red Light foods.

Think of a snack cracker on a plate. How long would it take to decompose? Granted, the stomach provides digestive enzymes to assist in the breakdown process, but the difference is still clear. A processed cracker lacks the digestive efficiency of a natural apple.

It's not as simple as saying Green Light foods are good and Red Light foods are bad. Green Light foods are simply better. They provide more nutrition and digestion efficiency. Of course, digestion varies from one person to another. How healthy is your digestive tract? Do you have acid reflux, irritable bowel syndrome (IBS), chronic constipation, Celiac's, Crohn's disease, or colitis? When away from home, do you hopscotch from one public restroom to another?

People with digestive troubles find Red Light foods even harder to digest. Poor digestion has a powerfully negative impact on health. On the flip side, a healthy digestive tract reflects overall good health. The relationship between what we eat and wellness is not a new concept.

Thomas A. Edison predicted, "The doctor of the future will give no medicine, but will interest her or his patients in the care of the human frame, in proper diet, and in the cause and prevention of disease." My guess is that Mr. Edison was a Green Light food kind of guy.

UNIQUELY ME, UNIQUELY YOU

The insides of our bodies are as unique as the outsides. We each digest and process food differently. I believe my husband has the digestive tract of a goat. He eats what he wants, when he wants, with nary a cramp or hiccup. Other than that nagging bout of cancer many years ago, he's the picture of health.

Me? I've had digestive difficulties since I was eleven. Several factors contribute to my condition (there's rarely one trigger). I believe a preteen trip to the dentist started my relationship with irritable bowel syndrome (IBS). What I call "the intestinal tornado" began about the same time as my first dental fillings — my introduction to the toxin, mercury.

Mercury is the second most toxic element on Earth (next to plutonium); yet, it's still used by dentists. Proven cases of heavy metal toxicity (from both dental amalgams and vaccines) currently have some medical professionals shying away from its use. Lawsuits speak louder than logic.

Debates about the link between vaccines and autism rage on, yet some facts stand firm. The incidence of autism has increased dramatically and so has the number of required vaccines. My oldest child had only a few vaccines required as a toddler, and by the time my youngest child was born, three times as many vaccines were recommended. While a vaccine may not *cause* autism, each individual child's health factors (i.e., genetics, immune system impairments, tendencies toward food allergies, frequent use of antibiotics, poor diet, compromised digestive system, etc.) should be considered when deciding to introduce any medications or vaccines.

Removing heavy metals from the body is a complex endeavor. Although methods vary and authorities differ on the approach, most agree that nutritional deficiencies should be remedied first. It's probably a good idea to strengthen your immune system by repairing nutritional problems before seeking heavy metal detoxification programs.

IBS and other digestive disorders are also affected by other factors such as food intolerances (and one's inherited tendency toward them), hormones, stress, environmental conditions, even posture and tight clothing.

Fibrofolk are ultra-sensitive to smells, sounds, and bright lights. A momentary whiff of toxic cleaning products or perfumes can trigger a migraine. Sensitivity to external toxins is common. Doesn't it stand to reason that this ultra-sensitive tendency applies to what we internalize, too?

External toxins are as problematic as internal ones. Protect your personal environment. Limit exposure to external chemicals, including chemical-laden health and beauty products, detergents, scents, lawn and fertilizer products, and cigar/cigarette smoke. Become more aware of your external surroundings.

Internally, find out what's eating you by taking a look at what you're eating (and internalizing unintentionally). Dental amalgams can leak heavy metals directly to your bloodstream, wreaking havoc with the central nervous system. Removing old mercury fillings is unwise unless done by a qualified holistic dentist. Check referral sources such as the International Academy of Oral Medicine and Toxicology[9] before allowing any dentist to remove fillings from your teeth.

Take a serious look at the foods you consume. Focus on foods suspected of causing irritation. Begin with a simple elimination diet (see further details in the Elimination Diet section later in this chapter). Eliminate a suspected food group for a period of time and analyze the results. Do you feel better? Learn to listen to your body; listen to both subtle and obvious indicators. Look for clues. Become your own food detective. How do you feel when you reintroduce an eliminated food? Here's an abridged symptoms list to help with your analysis:

_____ Sleepy
_____ Gurgly
_____ Bloated
_____ Headachy
_____ Gassy
_____ Intestinal discomfort (constipation/diarrhea)
_____ Moody/angry
_____ Itchy eyes/nose/skin

9   (IAOMT) http://www.iaomt.org/ [accessed 02/01/10]

_____ All of the above
(see more symptoms in the Elimination Diet section)

There's no denying that we often crave the foods that cause us the most intestinal grief. Food can be our enemy or our ally. It's better to work *with* food than *against* it. Unlike other addictions, abstinence from all foods isn't an option. We have to eat, so why not forge a truce?

ℬ

Making healthy food choices isn't easy. Nutritionists might disagree on which ingredients are best, but everyone seems to agree on the worst. These two items consistently top the charts for worst ingredients: trans fats and high fructose corn syrup (HFCS) — the diabolical duo.

These ingredients have been linked to obesity, diabetes, heart disease, and cancer. Although relatively new food additives, the evidence against them is strong enough to garner warnings from the Food and Drug Administration.

Trans fats *increase* bad cholesterol and *decrease* good cholesterol. Not a happy thing. A simple way to differentiate between the two numbers is this: think of HDL as "high cholesterol" and LDL as "low cholesterol." In general, high HDL and low LDL numbers are desirable. Trans fats also increase your triglycerides and inflammation, contributing factors in chronic illnesses such as diabetes.

Trans fats are an unnatural dietary fat source scientifically engineered to reduce the weight (and, therefore, shipping costs) of oil. As a manufacturing bonus, the hydrogenation process also increases its shelf life.

The bottom line is money. Imagine picking up a gallon jug of vegetable oil. That same volume of artificially generated trans fat (a fluffy, air-whipped product) is significantly lighter. Reduced weight and longer shelf life are financially beneficial to mass-market bakeries. It increases their profit margins. So why should we expect unbiased dietary information from food manufacturers regarding the nutritive value of trans fats?

As already mentioned, trans fats can be present even in products marked "contains no trans fat." If you read "partially hydrogenated" anything in the ingredients, put down the product and walk away.

The good news is that healthy fats, such as omega-3s, provide vital nutrients — good for the heart and the brain. Omega-3s can be found in quality fish oil, cod liver oil, and krill oil. Healthy oils (i.e. coconut, flax, olive, etc.), when paired with vegetables, can reduce the risk of inflammatory diseases such as rheumatoid arthritis. *Don't remove all fats from your diet. Replace unhealthy fats with healthy ones.*

Natural fats are fundamental to a healthy diet and help us maintain a healthy weight. For this reason, *low fat diets do not work.* When it comes to fats, the key is what type and in what proportion. Read Dr. Mark Hyman's blogs[10] on the relationship between low fat diets and heart disease. Refer to Dr. Mercola's extensive articles on his super-searchable website.[11] Both doctors have written multiple best-selling books providing comprehensive information on nutrition.

Unlike fats, there is no "healthy" sweetener. They vary from tolerable to toxic. I use whole leaf stevia in my tea (or better yet, no sweetener at all). High fructose corn syrup (HFCS) is definitely nearer the toxic end, being a fairly recent addition to the American diet. In 1984, soda manufacturers switched from cane sugar to HFCS, fueling increased consumption.

The body doesn't process HFCS in the same way it does table sugar. Standard sugar (sucrose) is converted into energy, increasing the production of a hormone (leptin) that controls the appetite. At the same time, it reduces another hormone (ghrelin) that makes hunger go away. HFCS appears to have the opposite effect: Rather than quenching an appetite, HFCS stimulates it *and* leaves you feeling hungry. This topsy-turvy result sounds similar to how trans fats are metabolized, doesn't it? Both fake products fool the body into thinking something that isn't true.

There's no great mystery to the connection of HFCS and the obesity epidemic in America. HFCS has exploded into the food market as the only sweetener used in soft drinks. It's even found

---

10   Links available at http://www.drhyman.com/ [accessed 02/02/10]

11   http://www.mercola.com/ [accessed 02/02/10]

in "healthy" bottled products such as teas, salad dressings, and sports drinks. It lurks in packaged food items from granola bars to cough syrup. Some experts believe that simply eliminating trans fats and HFCS from the standard American diet could result in a significant reduction of weight-related diseases.

> "*Re-examine all you have been told.... Dismiss what insults your soul.* "
>
> —Walt Whitman

Trans fats contributed to my own sickness. At my poorest health, I ate little, but what I did eat was highly processed. Boxed, bagged, and canned foods were a daily staple, crackers a main entrée. I rarely ate sweets and thought I was doing the right thing. I now realize I ate foods that *caused* inflammation and then wondered why I was so swollen. I didn't comprehend the vicious cycle I had created with my food choices.

I can't claim ignorance now, so it's good riddance to HFCS and trans fats!

GOOD, BETTER, BEST

I'd like to create a cable TV game show featuring a host who saves innocent bystanders from unhealthy dining choices. It would provide dietary clues spooned in palatable doses like this: "Contestants, after reading the nutritional information for each of these drinks, which do you choose? This large, blended coffee drink or the whole fruit smoothie? The six-hundred-and-fifty-calorie coffee drink contains twenty five grams of fat with only traces of protein and fiber. Yes! The strawberry-banana smoothie with added flax is the better choice at only two-hundred-and-thirty calories and five grams of fat. Additionally, the smoothie provides a whopping eleven grams of protein and ten grams of fiber."

The show could finish off with a Grocery Cart Ambush bonus round. "What's hiding under your *National Inquirer*?"

Now *that's* reality TV.

Eating well is about making better food choices, more wow and nutritional bang for your buck. A large, well-known department store revolutionized marketing in the nineteenth century with its GOOD, BETTER, BEST philosophy. I believe this concept is just as applicable to dining tools as it is to power tools.

Each snack or meal provides us with an opportunity to make a healthy decision. I've used corn chips to demonstrate this concept to an audience. Reading from the label of a familiar chip brand, I stumble over some of the fifty-four artificial ingredients. A label from the second bag lists only seven ingredients. The third sample, from a local health food market, has three ingredients: corn, sesame oil, sea salt.

Which is the healthiest choice? You're right if you selected the food closest to its original state, just plain corn. It also happens to have the fewest ingredients. Of course, corn chips aren't "healthy," but the point is, the third example is the healthiest of the three.

Looking for fewer ingredients may be simplistic, but it's a good start toward healthier eating. You might as well make the healthiest choice possible with everything you eat. Experiment with fresher, healthier ingredients. Start this exchange with your favorite and most-eaten foods, expanding to the rest of your diet.

Notice the similarity between the GOOD, BETTER, BEST dining options and the chronic illness stages in my Breakfast Menu of Acceptance from Chapter Four. Like everything else in life, eating better is a process.

The first step is to begin reading labels. Pay attention to what you eat. That's GOOD, a giant leap forward toward better dietary choices.

We gain confidence as we increase our familiarity with fresh ingredients. Choosing healthier alternatives begins the BETTER phase. When dining out, ask the server how food is prepared and seek healthier substitutions. Review food-related news blurbs online, read nutrition and health books and magazines. Become an informed consumer. We have all the ammunition we need to wage food battles and win the war.

The BEST phase creeps up silently. It's possible to not notice the shift from trying to avoid junk food to not even missing it. Making healthier choices becomes routine, ordinary, second nature.

I thought the world would spin off its axis when I discovered bread, crackers, and pasta carried on guerrilla warfare in my digestive tract. Life was barely worth living without bagels. I was bitter; I felt deprived.

It took a long time to accept my dietary fate. I went through a mourning phase, feeling isolated and alone in my experience. After my protracted pity party, I went into a lengthy BETTER phase. I sought every bread alternative imaginable. I found recipes on celiac disease websites (wheat/gluten intolerance is common for fibrofolk) and experimented. I searched for gluten-free breads at health food stores and farmers' markets. I didn't plan on weaning myself from all bread products. It was evolutionary. I went from bagels and cereals, to pitas, wraps, and what I called hockey pucks (Hawaiian dry oat cakes). I clung to them like dietary lifelines to the past. My rewards of reduced pain and better digestion far outweighed any satisfaction bread had ever given me.

One day, I was struck by an absurd thought: *I don't miss bagels.* I didn't miss crackers, chips, or other baked goodies, either. I realized I no longer looked for bread substitutions at the market. I no longer considered them "missing."

I'd found so many foods to *add* to my diet (veggies and proteins) that I'd forgotten about what to remove. I traded "woe is me" for "yay me!"

I'd stumbled upon the BEST phase.

INFLAMMATORY REMARKS

Inflammation is the body's natural response to injury or illness. Unattended, it runs rampant. Inflammation spreads, causing tender joints and muscles. Inflammation is a symptom of, and a trigger for, autoimmune conditions.

When the delicate balance of bacteria in the digestive tract is compromised over time, one main symptom of internal inflammation is yeast proliferation. Candida (fungal overgrowth) has been called the invisible pandemic because it can exist unnoticed for years. By the time it's symptomatic, it's difficult to control.

Symptoms of candida overgrowth include fatigue, mental cloudiness, irritability, headaches, disorientation, anxiety, confusion, and depression.[12] Simple at-home tests can help determine if you

12 Don Colbert, M.D., author of *The Bible Cure for Candida and Yeast Infections*

have yeast overgrowth. Dr. Colbert's books provide authoritative and easy-to-read information. His pocket-sized candida booklet is only eighty-six pages long, yet powerfully informative.

The following are likely the main sources of inflammation: substances, both internal and external, that are toxic to the body, poor diet, stress, and food intolerances or allergies. No wonder there's a proliferation of fibromyalgia and autoimmune ills in this country.

I first tripped over the term "autoimmune" almost twenty years ago when researching potential hazards before a friend's breast augmentation surgery. I found repeated references to autoimmune disease and wondered at the connection with silicone implants. I now understand that anything foreign (plastic, chemicals, toxins, heavy metals) in the body can have disastrous results, impacting the central nervous system.

The unanswered question is why these foreign elements negatively affect only some. Heredity isn't the only factor and doesn't guarantee sickness or wellness. Still, that's a roulette wheel I don't care to spin. For my family and me, I avoid potential triggers for autoimmune reactions.

Incorporating healthy food habits, regular exercise, and stress management techniques into daily life provides inflammation-fighting benefits. It's no coincidence, therefore, that nearly every healing suggestion in this book leads to reduced inflammation and a healthier body and life.

෨

I once saw a digitally altered picture of Michelangelo's "David." It depicted him as an obese man, intended to graphically project what he'd look like in our contemporary, overindulgent society. His chiseled form gave way to a more, uh, gelatinous silhouette.

Having seen the original sculpture in person, I found this alteration a sacrilege, but it did get me thinking. What sculpts our bodies?

Basic nutritional biology explains that the food we eat is converted to energy. That energy is burned off through exercise and other daily physical expenditures. Calories consumed, but not used, are stored for future use.

Because a lot of "leftover" food is acidic, and, therefore, a threat to the body, it's converted into a safer form — fat. That's the body's way of protecting itself. Fat is stored for safekeeping and awaits the day it's needed. And waits and waits….

Unfortunately, when we make too many deposits and too few withdrawals, we build up a reserve of "leftovers." I bet you never thought of your body as a life-sized food-storage container! Tupper-Wear?

The good news is our sculpted bodies are *not* carved in stone. Unlike Italian marble, fat is a malleable, changeable element. Nutrition and exercise provide us the physical tools of the body-sculpting trade. Rather than reaching for a mallet and chisel, go for a green salad with roasted salmon and a brisk walk around the park. There's beauty in making healthy food choices. It may even be considered an art.

SWEET SATISFACTION

Most people tend to crave either sweet or savory foods. For me, there's no contest. Sweet wins over savory, hands down. Sugar tastes good, but it's definitely not good for me.

It's helpful to learn what sugar does to the body. Four major factors break down the epithelial layer of skin (especially in women): excessive sun exposure, alcohol consumption, cigarette smoking, and sugar consumption. These factors *speed up the aging process.* I'd rather speed up my metabolism than my aging.

Most people are surprised to learn of sugar's role in causing the "decay" or breakdown of our bodies. Excess sugars in the system can trigger glycation, which decreases the skin's supply of collagen and elastin. This decay happens internally and externally. While aging is inevitable, giving the process a turbo boost isn't desirable.

I witnessed this breakdown progression firsthand when I bought a pre-made salad of baby spinach, dried cranberries, candied walnuts, and vinaigrette dressing. Because it was "fresh," the slimy greens under the walnuts surprised me. The rest of the salad was pristine. I realized the sugar from the walnuts had accelerated the decaying process. How degrading!

Sugar assists in breaking things down (like skin elasticity). It also helps to make things grow (like tumors). When scientists want cancer cells to proliferate for study, they feed them sugar. Yes, the body is essentially one large Petri dish, so it's important to watch what foods we include in our life-long experiment.

I've greatly reduced my sugar cravings (by making healthier choices), but I still indulge my love for chocolate. Because I choose to include chocolate in my life, I've done a bit of palate retraining. Over time, I've acquired a preference for healthier dark chocolate. A little taste nearly every day keeps me from feeling deprived. I enjoy my treat far more now than I ever did when I ate more but did so mindlessly.

One afternoon at an import store, I compared the ingredients of scads of chocolate bars. I purchased many and divided them into single portions, putting them in the freezer. I enjoyed a summer of chocolaty experimentation. I sampled, tasted, savored, nibbled. I found my favorites and worked my way toward less-sweet varieties. I now prefer the darkest chocolate I can find with three or fewer grams of sugar per serving.

Because I prefer dark, rich chocolate (yes, I'm a chocolate snob), it's easy for me to pass on those containing cheaper ingredients. Milk chocolate now tastes too sweet and flavorless to me. It feels oily or waxy. I think poor quality chocolates (the foil-wrapped, stocking-stuffer types) taste like melted brown crayons. Blech.

I shared the results of this experimentation at a lecture on nutrition. As mentioned in the Introduction, that was a mistake. At the word "chocolate," I lost my audience. Afterward, I was peppered with questions — about my favorite chocolate brands.

I understand that desire. Simply put, chocolate makes me happy. I suspect that's the case for many. Healthy eating isn't about exclusion; it's about inclusion. *Include* nutrients that sustain both the body and soul. When we consume healthy, whole foods, cravings for less-healthy foods diminish. A taste is all we need. For me, the search to discover my favorite chocolate brand was half the fun. And finding it? Sweet success.

Speaking of "just a taste," did you know that a simple eight-ounce glass of fresh juice may contain as much as eight teaspoons of sugar? How could something so tasty and touted as healthy hold such an unpleasant surprise? Sure, it's the fruit type of sugar and not the table-sugar type, but it's still heart-pumping sugar.

Drinking juice is one of the quickest ways to unwittingly increase calorie intake. It also provides a deceptively short-lived sense of fullness. The sugar spike actually increases hunger, making you more likely to overeat later.

A better option is to consume the whole fruit: fewer calories, plus fiber. A strawberry "one hundred percent juice" box (eight ounce) in my fridge has one hundred and twenty calories. The equivalent weight in whole strawberries is fifty calories. It doesn't take a mathematician to see the disparity. And, of course, the whole fruit contains calcium as well as wonderful fiber, which stabilizes the release of sugar in your system. The juice contains neither.

Remember it this way: *the whole fruit and nothing but the fruit.*

POP CULTURE

Early on in my nutritional education, I attended a lecture by an articulate nutritionist I'll call Dr. Eatwell. She gave an enlightening speech on information new to me. Her digestive system charts were exciting. I felt like Elizabeth Taylor untying a ribbon from a Tiffany's box. This was something new, something applicable, something I could sink my teeth into.

Dr. Eatwell fielded this simple question. "Which is better, diet or sugared sodas?"

Her answer of "neither" started a revolution. A debate on the dangers of artificial sweeteners versus the detrimental affects of sugar raged. Seeking a clear winner, the crowd could not be appeased. Dr. Eatwell departed long before the last of the bickering throng.

Of course, Dr. Eatwell was right. No soda is good for you.

Sodas have replaced white bread as the number-one source of calories in the American diet. Things have changed dramatically since soda first appeared on the market. In 1921, American artist Norman Rockwell depicted young sweethearts innocently sharing a soda at a local Sweet Shoppe. Seriously. Two people, one mini-serving, two straws. That's roughly fifty-two calories each.

Nowadays, children drink from cups big enough to provide adequate housing for a family of goldfish. Standards have changed — and not for the better. A typical convenience store mega-mouthful drink contains sixty-four ounces at a whopping eight-hundred-forty calories.

Then there's the artificially sweetened variety. The adverse effects of artificial sweeteners are too many to mention. If you're unaware or unsure about how these chemical compounds react in your body, I encourage you to review the Resources section of this book. Contrary to what you hear, NO artificial sweeteners are healthy. They are neither natural nor made from sugar. Additionally, sweeteners aside, all sodas contain enough acidity to deteriorate tooth enamel.

So what to do?

Once you've decided to make positive nutritional changes in your diet, begin by eliminating sodas. Replace regular soda intake with clean, pure water. As we fill up with refreshing water, we naturally lose the craving for soda. For heavy soda drinkers, consider replacing every other one with the equivalent amount of water. Work toward eliminating sodas entirely. You'll soon notice how water quenches your thirst whereas sodas fuel it, making you thirsty (and hungry) for more.

> "*When diet is wrong, medicine is of no use. When diet is correct, medicine is of no need.*"
>
> —Ancient Ayurvedic Proverb

It does not happen overnight, but giving a soda addiction the boot is something the body will appreciate. In fact, a thank you note may appear the next time you step on a bathroom scale.

KID-FRIENDLY

Yes, "real" foods can be a real pain. They're prepared by hand, may need refrigeration, and are often less than portable. There's no Twinkie shelf life for a chopped tomato.

Real foods also can be messy, especially for little fingers. Obviously, chicken nuggets are easier for children to eat than chicken drumsticks, but who's the boss in your kitchen? Parents get to decide what to feed their children. Real chicken isn't always boring. Look for fun and healthy cookbooks at bookstores or libraries and try interesting recipes. You can even make your own baked chicken nuggets, if that's your desire.

Be proactive about making healthy decisions for your family. Look for Green Light foods to serve at home. Before long, children will find independence, making their own food choices. It's important to lay the groundwork now for your child's future. And there's no such thing as too late. Any time is a good time to incorporate healthy food choices.

Watching a few minutes of TV commercials demonstrates that healthy food isn't going to come looking for you. Make a grocery list of tasty, fresh foods and snacks and serve them at home. Besides improved health, the potential for fewer cavities and reduced medical costs will be your family's rewards.

READY TO RUMBLE

Do you wake up hungry? If there isn't a rumbly in your tumbly, there should be.

If you don't feel the urge to fill your tank when you wake, it's likely you ate too much the night before. We all know the credo, "eat breakfast like a king, lunch like a prince, and dinner like a pauper." But do we follow this royal advice? Skip breakfast and we're more inclined to overeat and snack the rest of the day.

First thing upon waking, drink at least sixteen ounces of water. Do this before eating or drinking anything else. Follow up with a filling breakfast (including complex carbohydrates and/or protein), a healthy lunch, and a light dinner. Include plenty of water throughout the day. Tea can also hydrate the body as long it does not have added caffeine, sugars, or artificial sweeteners. Keep snacking to a minimum. Limiting snacks and beverages (other than water) after dinner can also reduce or eliminate acid reflux symptoms, as well as allow better sleep.

Follow this game plan, and wake every morning ready to rumble!

ELIMINATION DIET – SOLUTIONS FOR FOOD TROUBLES

Some foods can be the source of great digestive trouble. So how can you tell? A simple blood test can check for more than two-hundred sensitivities. But if a doctor's visit is cost-prohibitive, don't stay in the dark. Your own elimination diet can help pinpoint "trouble" foods. Remove a suspected problem food from your regular diet for at least one week or as long as several months. Afterward, reintroduce it (sometimes called a food challenge) and note any adverse effects. Eliminate one food or several, but reintroduce them one at a time. Separate the reintroductions by at least one week.

When a food is reintroduced, watch for one or more of the following symptoms:

- Itchy eyes or nose
- Runny nose
- Increased phlegm in bronchial tubes
- Headaches and/or migraines
- Sleepy/foggy feeling
- Allergy or hay-fever-like symptoms
- Asthma/wheezing
- Rashes/eczema/acne/boils/hives
- Muscle/joint pain
- Elevated heart rate
- Low blood pressure
- Emotional disturbances
- Memory problems
- Halitosis
- Unpleasant body odor
- Digestive problems including gassiness, diarrhea, constipation

Foods most often connected to allergies or intolerances are: dairy products (including cheese), gluten/wheat products,[13] soy, eggs, nuts, corn and corn products, colas, shellfish, caffeine, processed foods (due to chemical additives, artificial sweeteners, flavorings, dyes, etc.), and chocolate.

There are many types of elimination diets, so find one tailored for your needs. From my experience, eliminations diets are not as hard as accepting the results. I learned to simply stay away from inflammation-causing foods, but acceptance didn't take place overnight.

Feeling better leads to improved health. For me, removing

---

13   See http://www.celiac.com/ for their Unsafe Food List found under Popular Articles [accessed 01/10/10]

wheat and gluten made such a dramatic improvement in my joints (particularly my hands), that I no longer needed the arthritis gloves I'd worn for years. Abstaining from inflammation-causing foods is good for you and everyone around you. Food sensitivities also can cause negative emotional and mood flare-ups with or without physical symptoms.

In general, eating foods that are not processed (whole, natural foods), is called "eating clean" and is recommended for the majority of your meals. Some say that an eighty/twenty balance is healthy. Eating clean eighty percent of the time leaves a twenty percent "grace" factor for foods that may be not-so healthy.

The good thing about education is that it can never be taken away. Once you know what foods work with you rather than against you, the culinary world is your oyster. That is, as long as you don't have an intolerance to shellfish.

"In order to change we must be sick and tired of being sick and tired."

—Unknown

Chapter 6

Trade sick and tired for fit and inspired.

Exercise is how I put my wellness plans into action. Once I understood my nutritional deficits, my physical ones became more obvious. I'd like to say I began exercising with caution and care, but I didn't. I jumped in with both feet and never looked back.

❧

Exercise. Simply repeating the word aloud can burn calories —when accompanied by an involuntary shudder.

Exercise has not always been my friend. I'm not a fitness fanatic and have never been remotely athletic. I've had spells of being fit and spells of having them. I'll admit to following more than a few fitness fads: jogging in a silky, ice-blue, homemade track suit, aerobics with fuzzy crayon-colored leg warmers, and "gettin' jiggy wit it" in ridiculously clingy leotards. My consistency with a workout routine was as fickle as the fashions.

Shortly after my diagnosis, I read that regular exercise helps to manage chronic illness symptoms. I was to consider exercise as "doctor-prescribed." That sounded like real commitment. Ugh.

How could I get fit when I could barely stand? I needed a cane to compensate for balance issues, to navigate open spaces such as parking lots, and for standing in long lines. My cane signaled the beginning of the end of my mobility.

I didn't believe that exercise would work, but when a "women only" gym opened up nearby, it seemed like kismet. I had to at least look like I was trying. I appeared proactive, but I knew different. I joined the gym to *prove* it wouldn't work. I suffered from constant pain and dizziness. How could I exercise? I peeked inside at the workout machines, balance balls, resistance bands, and weighted hula hoops. My cane was not a gym-friendly accessory.

I joined anyway.

Expecting to fall (planning for failure *is* Norwegian optimism), I positioned myself within reach of something solid. Staggering on the treadmill like Captain Jack atop the Black Pearl, my simple goal was to stay upright. I gripped the weight machines for dear life and prayed for the room to stop spinning. Collapsed into a manageable size, my cane kept my gym bag company in a cubby space.

Time flew by. I worked out six days a week and chatted with everyone around me. I shared experiences, family news, and plans. Sometimes, I even forgot I was sick. I found myself building relationships as much as building muscle. Before long, a staff member informed me that my identity there as "that woman with fibromyalgia" had changed to "that woman who comes every day." And my dizziness? It fluttered away when I focused on other things. I'm not saying it went away because I ignored it, but I believe that my increased core strength and stamina healed many of my symptoms, including dizziness.

Along the way, I met great women and developed sustaining relationships centered on the primary concept of healthier living. I balanced my work, home, and gym life, putting fibromyalgia symptoms on a back burner.

Fibromyalgia was no longer the focus of my life.

I found a combination of cardio workouts and weight-lifting effective for rebuilding wellness, but I wanted weight loss, too, especially below the belt. I wanted to focus on lower-body workouts in an effort to accelerate results.

The staff at the circuit training center encouraged me to make full use of the gym, working out both upper and lower body as well as cardio training. I followed directions, but considered the upper-body workouts a nuisance. I didn't want buff biceps.

About six months later, I tried a new way to use a deltoid pull machine (designed to work the shoulder muscles). I sat on it backwards, facing away from others. I pulled the overhead bars up and down as the instructor showed me and heard whispers behind my back. A woman asked the instructor how she could get trapezius and deltoid muscle definition across her upper shoulders like "that lady." Muscle definition, me?

The upper body workouts were more effective than I realized. I conceded that I was physically stronger, but I'd also gained inner strength. An irreplaceable confidence. Strengthening my entire body gave me unexpected stability; my balance issues became a thing of the past. The benefits of exercise far exceeded my expectations, and I realized this:

Strengthening the core of my body strengthened the core of me.

Does it matter that I started my fitness journey with stubbornness? Does it matter that I planned to prove it wouldn't work? Of course not. Ignorance can be useful; as a motivator, it's highly underrated.

I unwittingly proved that my body has the power to heal. I learned to trust my body and my inner voice when it came to physical fitness. I learned when to push myself and when to pull back and conserve my energy.

Self-awareness and the opportunity to break a little sweat was one of the best gifts I've ever given myself. Your gift is wrapped and ready to open. What are you waiting for?

AFTERBURN

For those of us with chronic illness, new routines are difficult. Even more so if we're in pain, and the routine involves movement. Working my way into working out was neither quick nor easy.

About four months into my new workout regimen, I was still in pain and didn't know which way to go. I saw improvements in some symptoms like sleep, energy, and digestive troubles, but pain still clung to my bones. Like being lost in a cave, I didn't know whether to reverse and back out or keep moving forward. Each day, saying "see you tomorrow" to my new friends at the gym kept me committed.

I'd previously done sporadic workouts at home, but this everyday routine was tough. I aggressively pursued improvements in the number of repetitions done on each machine and tracked my progress. I felt if I pushed myself a bit harder, I'd break free from the pain that gripped my back, neck, and shoulders.

Most journeys reach a point of no return — a point at which

we weigh efforts exerted against efforts yet to come. Things look hazy. I didn't know if my increased pain was real or imaginary. I wondered about a Herxheimer Reaction (feeling worse before feeling better). Was I progressing or regressing?

Sensing no clear answer, I kept going. I dropped weight (encouraging, yes), but, what about my fibromyalgia? Some days I made it through my workout hardly breaking a sweat. Others, I barely kept up. It made no sense. The gym stayed consistent, the machines, timing, routine. The only variable seemed to be my personal energy. I tracked my fatigue and pain levels, finding a direct correlation between pain and the success of my workouts.

Back then, I didn't know anyone else with fibromyalgia. I tried to make sense of my kooky condition on my own. Now, I'm glad for what I didn't know. If I'd heard from any "fibromyalgia authority" (medical professional, author, etc.), that exercise might make things worse, I definitely would have quit. Instead, I slogged along in ignorance.

I also didn't know that sweating is a powerful detoxification tool. I was sweating out toxic wastes as well as toning and strengthening my body. Ridding the body of toxins can cause temporary side effects, such as headaches and joint and muscle pain. Had I known better, I could have slowed my pace a bit and increased my water consumption to mitigate the increased pain.

I'll admit, for the first four or five months, my gym visits fulfilled needs more social than physical. New friendships kept me going. I hadn't planned on it, but I found comfort, camaraderie, and encouragement in one location. Oh, yeah, with a little exercise thrown in.

At about the six-month mark, I realized my cane had taken up permanent residence in the trunk of my car. Even better, I'd lost fifteen percent of my starting body weight. Increased upper body strength, and the reduction of body fat, fatigue, and dizziness were the benefits. Gaining friends and personal confidence, bonuses.

But wait … there's more. Where did the all-encompassing pain go? The majority of it ebbed away almost unnoticed. How could something as fundamental as healthy eating and physical fitness have such dramatic results?

Diet and exercise. I was well on my way toward restoration.

HOW REVOLTING!

I have mutinous muscles. Or, at least I did have, before I began a regular exercise program. That was part of my baffling symptom list before my diagnosis. I appeared in good physical condition, yet, I spent far too many nighttime hours hobbling up and down my hallways, trying to loosen the cramps in my legs and feet. My muscles twitched all night as if I'd run marathons all day.

Sleep deprivation symptoms followed nights with charley horse stampedes. Doctors told me I exaggerated, that muscles don't cramp nearly every night. They had no answers, so I tried my own cures. I swallowed pills, applied lotions, took long, hot detox soaks. I tried potassium, magnesium, calcium, and manganese supplements. I ate bananas until I could swing from trees and glugged enough chalky white concoctions to stripe a football field. Nothing helped.

" Success is to be measured not so much by the position that one has reached in life as by the obstacles which he has overcome. "

—Booker T. Washington

My nighttime leg cramps only diminished as my daytime workouts increased. It turns out that muscles are designed for use. Like our brains, muscles are healthiest when stimulated and exercised. Regular exercise keeps toxins from taking up residence in the muscle fibers, and helps maintain healthy blood flow to surrounding tissues. When I think of toxins and bad stuff sticking to my muscles, I think of how threads, lint, and bits of dirt stick to the Velcro® on my kids' shoes. How effective is Velcro® when it's goobered up?

Speaking of goobers, muscles can also hold on to bad memories, emotions, and stress. Exercise releases tensions and is a great mood elevator. We know that "happy" endorphins are released during exercise; add stress reduction, and you can see why exercise is cathartic. Exercise provides physical *and* emotional benefits. Time spent exercising gives opportunity to clear the mind and think profound thoughts.

One thought struck me as I awoke from yet another night of

blissful slumber. The deeper I plunge into exercise, the deeper I sleep at night. I've found my ultimate circadian rhythm!

GET GOING, THEN GET LOST

If you like the outdoors, walking may be the exercise of choice for you. Leave running and jogging to those with pain-free joints; simply challenge yourself to a brisk pace.

If practicality keeps you indoors, you don't have to forgo fitness. Before spending money on DVDs or expensive equipment, review consumer comments online or ask friends for recommendations. Even better, borrow a video, weights, a stability ball, or resistance bands to see what feels right. What fitness education resources measure up at your local library or community center? Many cities offer a variety of low-cost classes, such as yoga, low-impact aerobics, tai chi, dance, stretching, aqua therapy, and Pilates.

Fitness DVDs are as proliferous as dandelions. Read the package descriptions and pay attention to the intended fitness levels. Beginners? Experts? Watch out for unrealistic goals or claims. Does a DVD promise to have you looking as you did in high school, or like a waif-thin celebrity? That may not be a good idea. Rent or borrow DVDs before you buy to decide if they're right for you.

I searched for fitness routines that could be adapted for those with physical limitations or restricted range of motion. There are exercise DVDs just for fibrofolk. The non-impact yoga moves of Fibroga[14] are designed specifically for those with limited mobility.

One piece of home gym equipment I couldn't do without, is a mini-trampoline or rebounder. I purchased one for about thirty dollars at a discount store several years ago and still use it almost daily. Who can't find fifteen minutes here or there to bounce around? It jostles stiffened muscles, and gets the blood flowing. Improved circulation helps reduce muscle spasms as well as overall pain. In only minutes of bouncing, I benefit from stress relief, too. A trampoline is beneficial for those with joint and muscle health issues. Shaking things up (gently) gets the heart pumping, and provides a great energy boost. It's even good for the brain! Purchase one with a stability bar or pole to help with balance.

---

14.   http://www.thegroveapproach.com/ [accessed 01/10/10]

I've often said living with fibromyalgia is like living with rigor mortis. In a "move it or lose it" fashion, muscles and tendons tighten up from disuse, and stiffness sets in quickly. To combat this tendency (besides jumping on the trampoline), I frequently roll my shoulders and move my head and neck. I never mind what the people behind me in theaters, auditoriums, or at church think. *Gotta keep movin.'*

After selecting favorite fitness activities, it's time to get lost. Lose yourself in nature, music, your own thoughts. Combine favorite mental activities with favorite physical activities. Do what's necessary to take a mental break from day-to-day frustrations. Get lost in thoughts that interest you, and get lost in the physical experience. Surfing, horseback-riding, rollerblading, gardening, biking, nature walks, yoga, and tai chi in the park are all examples of this ideal mental/physical combination.

Don't happen to live close to the beach or mountains? Do what moviemakers do. Make a soundtrack for your exercise routine. Walking down a crowded suburban street with Vivaldi's *Four Seasons* on your MP3 player can mentally take you to the canals of Venice or the forests of Germany. Movies use music and sounds to influence our thoughts and emotions. Manipulation turns to motivation when used with your own permission.

What music speaks to your soul? One man's cello is another man's Incan panpipe. Try classical while walking, hip-hop for weightlifting, and soothing nature sounds for tai chi or yoga. Switch things up. Creating a personalized soundtrack is one part of making your own exercise routine. Remember, when you customize your regimen to fulfill both your physical *and* emotional needs, you're more likely to follow through.

Everyday life includes a lot of "haftas," like working and caring for family. When exercise becomes a "wanna" instead of a "hafta," you've crossed the border into the realm of a healthier you. Recognize this: by nurturing yourself, you're better equipped to nurture others.

TAI CHI AND ME

I've tried both yoga and tai chi. As with many classes, a good instructor makes all the difference. My tai chi instructor is not just good; she's amazing! For that and many other reasons, I've come to love tai chi. My favorite part involves tapping along the acupressure meridians, which wakes up and energizes parts of the body. I leave each class feeling rejuvenated and refreshed.

Instructor Melissa explains that tai chi is all about quieting the mind. She encourages us to "stop chasing shiny objects." Tai chi focuses thoughts into the present. By concentrating on the coordination of body movements, the mind lets go of other concerns.

Tai chi has numerous physical benefits. It employs a full range of motion: each body part is moved — slowly — to its natural extent and within its limitations. There's no hyperextending of knees or elbows, no straining, pressure, or impact to joints or muscles. Tai chi may look easy, but moving slowly with accuracy takes muscle control *and* mental focus. It also takes a concentration of breathing. Breathing with movement improves focus as well as blood flow. It becomes second nature to inhale in preparation to move, and exhale at the point of action.

Many tai chi moves involve a slow twisting of the spine; knees and shoulders diametrically opposed. This gentle move helps to relieve compression of the spaces between vertebrae in the spine, leading to better nerve communication. The spinal chord runs through the spine, acting as a superhighway of information from the brain to the body. Proper spinal alignment improves the spinal chord's ability to send and receive signals. Subtle twisting motions also help to adjust internal organs to their proper positions. I call these moves "chiropractic without the pop." Tai chi is a perfect complement to chiropractic treatment as it helps the body hold proper alignment.

It's important to extend muscles and ligaments in ways uncommon to daily living. Most of us lead fairly sedentary lives. When was the last time you rotated your entire arm in circles like a slow-mo softball pitcher? That shoulder rotator cuff needs movement. Moving little-used muscles and joints improves strength, elasticity, and blood flow. What about your neck and shoulders? A simple exaggerated shrug relieves pressure on your upper spine and neck. Instructor Melissa renamed one favorite qigong move the Tin Man. The slow, rhythmic, side-to-side motion "lubricates" the knees, hips, waist, and shoulders. It does so simultaneously, or "all in one swell foop."

Fibrofolk are particularly susceptible to head, neck, and shoulder pain. It's reflexive and second nature to protect these areas by immobilizing them. Yet, maintaining a stiff and awkward position has disastrous, lasting effects. Besides throwing off the body's natural alignment, it trains the muscles to reinforce the odd pose, making it difficult to move naturally. Tai chi *strengthens and lengthens* the muscles, thereby deepening the healing process. From hand/eye coordination to developing balance, tai chi treats the body from head to toe.

A pinched and tight body holds secrets. Movement allows the body to let them go.

As with any worthwhile investment, it takes time to reap the many benefits of tai chi. Obvious physical benefits may come easily, but the subtle stress-relieving aspects, less so. Be patient while learning to tune out your busy life and tune in to a healthier way of thinking. Tai chi can't be "phoned in." You have to pay attention and stay present to follow the intricate, flowing movements. After completing a complex set of Twenty Four Form moves, Instructor Melissa often says, "I bet you weren't making a mental grocery list while we did that!"

Tai chi combines breathing techniques with mental focus. Corral your thoughts long enough to complete the class, and you leave feeling physically and emotionally refreshed. The long-lasting benefits buoy you throughout the rest of the day. Additionally, tai chi improves digestion, focus, immune system function, and sleep. I sum it up this way: tai chi calibrates my internal compass.

BRAIN TRAINING

Lessons learned in tai chi can be carried through to other workouts. Being present is a difficult skill for linear thinkers like me. My mind often sprints ahead to my next task, preventing me from being present in my current one.

If I'm not fully present, mentally, I don't get the full benefit of the exercise. When I want maximum benefits, I turn *off* the TV and refrain from reading while on the treadmill or elliptical trainer.

Instead, I think about each muscle group, feeling it expand and contract. It seems counterintuitive when I could be multi-tasking, but why do each task halfway? If I'm spending the time to exercise, I want to gain the full benefit from it. This is *purposeful exercise*; my mind working in cahoots with my muscles for the greater good.

Yes, the body *does* listen to the mind.

I'm not blessed with the meditative gene. I work hard to quiet the busy thoughts Instructor Melissa appropriately calls, "monkey chatter." I'm thankful for the contemplative aspects of tai chi, including methodical breath flow. Learning to breathe deeply (shallow breathing is common for fibrofolk) takes practice, but provides both emotional and physiological benefits.

Aptly named, deep breaths are called "cleansing breaths." Why not start now? Breathe in deeply through the nose, and exhale slowly through the mouth. That's it. Put your mind to it, and you've already mastered two vital tenants of exercise.

SOMETHING TO TAP INTO

While I love tai chi, I'm always looking for additional methods to augment my fitness routines. My sister mentioned a "tap" video and, thinking it would be similar to tai chi, I checked it out.

I couldn't have been more wrong, yet right on. I found Teresa Tapp, a fitness guru, and her methodologies blew my socks off. Her low-impact/high-intensity moves blend with aerobic activities in a seamless physical flow. Her methods and philosophies are geared to help condition people with illnesses such as high-blood pressure, diabetes, and autoimmune disorders. Done properly, her routines put little to no pressure on joints. In fact, she's developed rehabilitation moves geared specifically for those with limited mobility.

Her fifteen minute video, *Basic Workout Plus*, has been a staple in my exercise routine for many years. I did a lot of research before falling in love with Teresa's philosophies. They make sense to me. Some of her stances and positions feel and look goofy, but I trust her education, experience, and intent. Her website[15] offers free video clips of exercises to try before you buy. (You'll also find many success stories to preview.)

---

15.   http://www.t-tapp.com/ [accessed 02/02/10]

Too many exercise video ads make unrealistic claims about the body you'll achieve when you buy, buy, buy. Theresa Tapp's methods are tried, true, honest. They really do work. It's success the old-fashioned way with a modern twist. Yes, you'll sweat. Yes, you'll work hard. But here's the best part: You'll get there lickety-split.

Her experience as an exercise physiologist led her to develop specific move combinations that increase the efficacy of each workout. What that means is that you get the most value for your time and dollars spent. You burn the most calories in the shortest amount of time. The results are proven and lasting, not a quick fix with temporary results.

T-tapp exercises are simply effective *and* fast.

THEME-STREAMS

After incorporating exercise into my life, I noticed common threads in my day-to-day experiences. Ideas wound through my conscious and subconscious like rivers of awareness. I call them *theme-streams.*

Some of these themes include tapping, cross-lateral movements, prioritizing, spinal communications, mind/body connection, focus, balance, and the act of choosing.

The "choosing" theme seeped in last, but became primary in importance. It just took me a while to get it. Instead of thinking about what I *couldn't* do, I began to focus on what I *could* do. I focused on choosing goals rather than on noticing obstacles. Along the way, obstacles lost their hold on me.

I found time to exercise regularly when I decided it was a health priority. Treating it as if doctor-prescribed makes good sense. I'll admit a health crisis sharpened my focus, but isn't that what crises do? There's nothing like an emergency to crystallize your sense of priorities. Choice is active thought. I *choose* to take care of my health, and I *choose* to make it a priority.

Tapping and cross-lateral movements also are common theme-streams in healing. Cross-lateral movement is the act of moving one side of the body while engaging the opposite side of the brain. Multiple examples exist in tai chi, qigong, dance, T-Tapp exercises, and Meridian Tapping Technique (more on MTT in Chapter Seven).

Activities combining mind and body have profound healing affects. Do you want to fire up your brain activity and improve hand and eye coordination? Play Ping-Pong! A highly competitive sport in some countries, Ping-Pong can even be aerobic. What about tetherball? It's one of the best examples of cross-lateral movement there is. Ping-Pong and tetherball are effective for healing and improving brain function.

When I realized the importance of self-care, I understood that I'd allowed my "good" health to slip away. A misalignment of priorities led me to make poor choices. I put my physical and emotional needs last. I've learned to strike a balance between my own needs and the needs of others.

> " *It is exercise alone that supports the spirits, and keeps the mind in vigor.* "
>
> —Marcus T. Cicero

Like a pendulum, you may find yourself swinging to the opposite extreme when you start to feel better. You go from never thinking of your needs to only thinking of them. If your needs reside prominently on the front burner, you may resent giving up that premier status. I read a blog post for a "recovered" fibromyalgia person who said she needed seven hours of every day for self-care. She managed her chronic illness symptoms with a daily routine of yoga, meditation, tai chi, massage, and long walks. I'm happy for her, and it sounds like a great life. But, I'm not jealous. That routine works for her, but wouldn't work for me. I have family, work, and other responsibilities that would make that lifestyle impossible.

The key is finding the right balance — for you. Once you decide to make wellness a priority, it's up to you to choose how to prioritize the rest of your life.

HOW SWEDE IT IS

When it comes to exercise, I'm often asked, "What's better, aerobics or weight training? Treadmill or elliptical? Aqua fitness or Pilates?"

My answer is always the same: *fartlek*.

The literal interpretation of this Swedish word is *speed play*. Swedes long ago discovered that the key to ultimate physical conditioning is to alternate activities. Athletes who practice fartlek change the speed and intensity of their workouts, keeping their bodies in a constant state of "what's next?" Fartlek, the antithesis of predictability, is often found in the conditioning routines of Olympians and professional athletes. I prefer to generalize its meaning to fit all forms of exercise. Everyone's exercise routine can use a little fartlek now and then.

Just as there's no one-size-fits-all diet, exercise is also an individual experience. By changing speed and intensity of movements, your body burns more calories and works more efficiently.

What exercises or activities appeal to you? If you don't find a particular exercise fun or at least interesting, odds are you won't continue. Keep looking for something you enjoy. For those with sore joints and fatigued muscles, water activities can prove beneficial (especially in natural lakes, rivers, and oceans). Prefer dry land? Walking is the ultimate fitness tool. Vary your speed to ensure a good workout. You can even jog at intervals (if able). But don't worry, just alternate speeds and work within your abilities.

By the way, you can alternate the "speed" of calorie intake, too. Calorie cycling is the dietary form of fartlek. The rule of thumb for weight loss is to eat fewer calories than needed to maintain your current weight. As the body becomes accustomed to the reduction, over time, the technique may lose its effectiveness. That's the all-too familiar weight-loss plateau. By decreasing (or even increasing) your calorie intake slightly, now and then, your body gets the jolt it needs to trigger further weight loss.

Exercise fartlek can be achieved in a variety of ways. If you workout on a treadmill, choose a setting that arbitrarily changes the pace and incline. For weightlifting, change the repetitions and the speed. It may seem contradictory, but slower repetitions increases intensity.

Once you've compiled a varied list of favorite activities, shuffle the order from time to time. Periodically select the less-favorites. If you walk one day, lift weights another. The key is to consistently challenge your body in new and healthy ways. Muscles have memory, so doing the same exercise over and over eventually ceases to provide the same benefits.

If the term *fartlek* doesn't grab you, might I suggest Tesla Training? In the late 1800s, Nikola Tesla pointed out that Edison's direct current method of transporting electricity loses lots of energy as it moves through wire. Edison wasn't amused. Today, Tesla's alternating current (A/C) method is industry standard. Tesla discovered that by alternating electrical currents, he increased the efficiency, speed, and distance of transmission.

Similarly, alternating exercise routines reduces energy loss and maximizes results. It allows the body to recoup from the use of one muscle group while engaging another. It incorporates the mind and body as creativity is needed to cope with new and ever-changing methods of training.

So what if Tesla wasn't a Swede? It apparently didn't stop him from thinking like one.

THE EYES HAVE IT

When it comes to muscle strength, the eyes have it. Of the twelve cranial nerves that control the entire body, half are solely dedicated to the eyes. Eye exercises should be part of your regular exercise routine.

Instructor Melissa had severe vision problems post brain tumor surgery. By including eye/vision exercises with her martial arts routines, she restored her vision to pre-surgery normal. She incorporates simple eye exercises into all of her classes.

When stretching your body, include your eye muscles. Look as far to the left as possible, then to the right. While holding your head still, look up and then down. I've personally found improvement in visual acuity and relief from nighttime eye strain when I'm consistent with eye muscle exercises. Eye movements are also a part of MTT (Meridian Tapping Technique) and have proved beneficial in altering negative thought patterns.

For an overview on basic exercises, online sources such as WikiHow[16] and Hanford Department of Energy[17] may prove helpful. Ask your trusted optometrist or ophthalmologist for suggestions on books or DVDs. You can't be too careful.

How important is your vision? Isn't it worth finding out how

---

16.   http://www.wikihow.com/Exercise-Your-Eyes/ (click on How to Exercise Your Eyes) [accessed 02/02/10]

17.   http://www.hanford.gov/amh/eye/index.html/ [accessed 01/31/10]

to maintain it? It's easier to keep your eye on the prize, when your eyesight is the best it can be.

THE SCALES OF JUSTICE

How often should you step on the bathroom scale? Responses to that question vary from "daily" to "never." The issue of "weighing in" sparks as much controversy as topics such as religion and politics. Everyone claims to have the real scoop.

We can agree, however, that weighing is an easy way to monitor weight-loss progress or health management. Other tools may be more accurate, but for the average John or Jane "Dough," the bathroom scale dictates victory or success. At least, that's what I thought.

After becoming a regular at the gym and sustaining my weight-loss goals for nearly a year, I heard a podcast message that was music to my ears. A fitness expert said, "I've thrown away my bathroom scale. After all, don't you *know* when your pants get snug?"

I embraced this idea whole hog. I was in peak physical condition, eating well, and exercising regularly. What more could a number on a scale tell me? I felt unleashed from numeric bondage. Free. FREE!

I was unleashed from bondage and from the truth. Within six months, my weight crept up alarmingly, *without* my knowledge. I realized it when I failed to slip gracefully into a pair of old jeans. I yanked them on halfway and said, "Hey, what gives?"

My dog's stare implied, "Not denim."

What a mystery. I worked out four to six days a week, stuck to a healthy diet, and still gained weight. Why?

I wish I'd known this: By the time your clothing feels uncomfortable, you may have already gained between ten and fifteen pounds. I also didn't know about the importance of varying exercise and nutrition routines. I didn't understand fartlek. I've learned that weighing myself regularly is an essential tool in my health-maintenance arsenal. It's vital for everyone — the naturally thin, the not-so-naturally thin, and the rest of us.

Weighing is only one measurement factor, but it's the easiest to do consistently. Strategically measuring your body provides a better indication of overall progress, but as with other things, it's only as effective as the follow-through. I usually measure myself at the beginning of a new exercise plan, but forget to re-measure later.

So, bring the scale back from it's banishment in the closet. Some experts say daily weighing is important, others suggest weekly. Or, settle for something in-between. You decide.

When you do weigh, don't fret about the small swing in numbers. Depending on your weight, that swing can average from two to four pounds, maybe more. Instead, save the worry for when your weight creeps over what's a normal "high" number for you.

Weighing yourself regularly gives you the power to take action and the wisdom to know when to do so.

If you know your average weight, a tip of the scale tips you off to weight gain. Getting rid of small upswings in weight (eliminating liquid pounds before they turn into solid pounds) is much easier.

Exercise is a great moderator for weight, but it's less effective without healthy eating. For the most part, I eat "healthy" after exercise so I don't "waste" my efforts. I'm always amazed to see people leave the gym and immediately purchase high-calorie coffees and smoothies. The calories they burned in exercise probably doesn't compare to what will be consumed.

If you are eating healthier, drinking more water, increasing exercise, and reducing stress in your life, it's likely that you're also losing weight (if you had it to lose). A scale won't tell you how to stay healthy, but it will help to keep you on track.

PAINSTORMING IDEAS

The fitness world is full of catch phrases. Motivational platitudes are designed to influence our spending, but do they alter our beliefs about exercise?

"No pain, no gain" *sounds* like it should be true. It does take effort to make progress, but exercising to the point of pain isn't beneficial for anyone, especially fibrofolk. Our pain indicators are already catawampus, so who needs to add more pain on purpose?

I've mentioned the strenuous exercise routine I adopted after my fibromyalgia diagnosis. By choosing frequent and intense workouts, I didn't follow conventional wisdom or actually any wisdom. The more pain I felt, the harder I pushed. My will was at cross purposes with my body. Not a good thing.

Because I'm stoic, stubborn, and tenacious, I pressed on, fighting my way through the pain. I could have achieved the same results — in a safer manner — by applying patience. I should have reduced the intensity of my workouts as my pain increased. I should have listened to my body when symptoms flared and exercised accordingly. I was correct in my dogged pursuit of fitness, but incorrect in practice.

I now know that fibrofolk have to listen to what their energy or pain level tells them. The body does have the final say. The general rule is to stop any exercise or movement *before* you feel pain. Yes, that's a lot like telling a roofer to stop the hammer mid-swing before it hits his thumb. But consider this; a skilled roofer hits his thumb less than his apprentice.

Through experience, we can learn to anticipate the signs before the crash. We can develop our own "sick sense." Putting mine into practice, I avoid activities or environments that cause symptom flares. I don't always miss hitting my thumb with the hammer, but, with time and practice, I can drastically reduce the frequency of injury.

When it comes to exercise, listen to your body's signals. Sometimes it's pull back and at other times, forge ahead. Obey the body if it says *take it easy today.* You may need a little extra nurturing ... but, be sure to get right back on track. Beware of the voice that says, "Skip the gym and go shopping." That's not nurturing. Working out to the point of muscle fatigue is good. But *how* fatigued is the question.

Moving forward through pain isn't easy. It's no wonder fibrofolk find it difficult to work with fitness trainers. We can't blame them for not understanding our physical limitations when we don't always "get it," either. Some days we're one step ahead of our condition and others, two steps behind. That's the fickle finger of fibro.

And then there's the problem of feeling good. Too good. That's when we overdo it. It's tempting to grab a ladder and paint that stained ceiling. And while we're buying more paint, why not stop off at the grocery store, too? This scenario rarely turns out well. The "overdoing it" tendency doesn't typically spill over to exercise. Feeling good leads to more trips to the mall than to the gym.

For many of us, lack of exercise is a major factor in unwanted weight gain. Thus begins a "chicken and egg" cycle. We don't exercise because we're in pain, which leads to weight gain, which leads to additional pain.

I encourage fibrofolk to simply move. Begin today. Find exercise routines that meet your needs and stick to them. The only way out of chronic pain is to *start somewhere*. Start an exercise plan. Increase physical activity in all areas of your life. Surround yourself with encouraging people, read encouraging books and magazines. Focus your thoughts on success and improved health.

And don't forget to breathe. Breathe deeply, and *choose* when and where to begin your fitness future.

LEVEL: BEST

I'm often asked, "How do I know if I'm working out hard enough?"

Ideal exertion levels vary as widely as those who exercise. Some fibrofolk can run miles without breaking a sweat; others feel winded tugging on the sports bra. It's a matter of fitness, not weight or age.

One indicator of fitness is heart rate. There are lots of fancy (read: expensive) gadgets to help track heart rates while exercising. Some elliptical and treadmill machines monitor it automatically. Don't be shy about asking gym staff for assistance. That's what they're there for.

If you prefer gadget-free options, here's a simple (i.e. more practical than scientific) method. Exercise to the point of feeling a bit winded. If it feels like it would be hard to carry on a conversation, that's the level you're looking for. At that point, back off just a bit and continue. That's your peak target rate. It's not important to stay at that pace for long or even work out to that level every time. It's a personal benchmark. That pace is what's good for you, and where you're working at your level best.

Another consideration is the time of day to work out. Why push to exercise at daybreak if that's when your knees and hip joints feel as if they're lined with fish-tank gravel? Maybe planning a crockpot dinner ahead of time allows you to hit the gym after work instead. Squeezing fitness into a busy life takes compromise. Learning to make it a priority takes practice. Respectfully set aside time to exercise. Think of it as self-care.

I'm fortunate to have found a healthy balance of work and physical activities, but it took time to figure out. If your Window of Well feels painted shut, try prying it open with a little self-analysis. Think about what priorities you wish to set, and align your goals accordingly.

In the past, my priorities were not aligned with my goals. It took a shift in thinking to realign them. I'm older and wiser, now.

Isn't that better than simply being older?

GAME PLAN

The recipe for exercise success is a lot like, well, a recipe. Do you have the ingredients you need? DVDs? Check. Gym membership? Check. Running shoes and weights? Check. Check.

But what happens if you don't use a recipe? If you put flour, yeast, and eggs into your pantry, I doubt you'd open the cabinet doors expecting to find bread. What do you expect from your physical fitness "ingredients" if you don't put them into action? You probably own videos, various equipment, gym memberships, etc., but, without a recipe, your exercise plan falls short every time.

"Change your thoughts and you change your world. *"*
—Norman Vincent Peale

Making an exercise recipe takes brain retraining. Instead of thinking in general terms, *I'll get fit someday*, be specific. Plan for specific results. Begin today.

Set a firm start date and stick to it. Don't give credence to negative thinking, i.e., gym time will take over my life; I'll become too sore to workout; I'll embarrass myself. Recipe results depend on follow-through. The same goes for exercise.

To make exercise a priority, employ user-friendly visual tools:

LISTS: Compile lists of exercise options you plan to try. For motivation, post them where you're likely to see them.

CHARTS: Chart your progress, including the types of exercise and frequency.

CALENDARS: Track your alternating weekly or monthly exercise schedules.

JOURNALS: Keep a written diary of your thoughts, progress, achievements, plans, goals, etc.

Written accountability ensures follow-through and success. Charting progress is a good way to challenge yourself and provide visual cues for rewards. Surround yourself with motivating messages. Food and exercise diaries can be particularly effective. Writing down what you eat and how much you move may prove more enlightening than you think.

Your fitness recipe should include about thirty minutes of exercise at least three times a week. Choose a variety of exercises and change your routine frequently. Give yourself time to see if you really enjoy a new activity. When you're physically challenged, it's easy to give up fast, thinking it's not "right" for you. Does that sound familiar? Instead, think about what *exactly* doesn't feel right? Is it the actual activity or the intensity? Is it too strenuous? Can the moves be adapted to suit your limitations? There may be outside factors such as the instructor, time of day, or the location. These can be changed. Try exercising at different times of day, or break thirty-minute workouts into two or three shorter sessions.

Sorry, but it won't help to try something once and say, "I proved it. Exercise doesn't work for me." If a workout is too strenuous or causes too much soreness, back down on the intensity — but don't stop!

Just because you haven't found the right way to work out doesn't mean you can't work out.

Be persistent. You'll find at least one activity you can live with, if not love. I've witnessed it over and over — moving the body on a consistent basis *will* make you feel better. I've even seen that "can live with" feeling turn into unabashed love.

Give a new exercise workout at least a two-month trial period (stop, of course, if you feel the exercise is harmful in any way). I try to give any new exercise routine about four months to judge its benefits.

Some exercise experiences prove less than successful. I once continued taking a particular yoga class much longer than I should have. Because yoga is a healing exercise, I believed it would improve my mobility. It didn't. At first, I thought I imagined increased joint and muscle pain. I felt more bruised than normal. Then, my wrists became so tender, it was hard to type (my livelihood). The yoga instructor said I was healing, not hurting, so I continued. I struggled through one painful pose after another (especially *downward dog*) for three months before finally giving up.

Yoga isn't supposed to hurt. Ever. There are many types (i.e. restorative yoga) that focus specifically on healing. In this case, it was the wrong kind of yoga and the wrong teacher for me. She didn't teach proper body mechanics (how external/internal factors affect the body's skeletal system) for someone with fibromyalgia. Even though I made modifications to the moves, the weight-bearing poses were held too often and for too long. My increased pain did not abate. I gave it a valiant try, but it wasn't for me.

Keep at something as long as you don't feel you're injuring yourself. Beneficial exercise tailored to *your* body *relieves* pain. It doesn't create it. Pursue fitness as you would any other desired goal. Listen to your muscles. You'll learn to sense if they're simply fatigued or feeling abused and overextended. Once you get used to a healthy, "tired muscle" feeling, you'll recognize it for the benefit that it is.

You might even get to the point of enjoying that exhausted-but-accomplished feeling after a workout. I know I do.

TODAY'S FORECAST: PARTLY SWEATY WITH SCATTERED PUSHUPS

How do you gauge the progress of an exercise program? If you wake up sore the next morning and say, "I guess that won't work for me," you're missing out. For most fibrofolk, every morning starts out with soreness. But post-exercise soreness is not fibromyalgia soreness. For one thing, exercise soreness is limited to the muscles recently exercised. Fibromyalgia soreness is that all-over feeling, as familiar as your old bathrobe.

Evaluating what I called "burnoff" in Chapter Three is a far better soreness monitoring tool.

Let me explain. At some point every day, fibromyalgia's Pain

Poncho shifts from debilitating to tolerable. When we wake, pain is usually at its worst. As we move, we loosen up; our joint and muscle pain begins to lessen. By paying attention, we can pinpoint when this happens. I wake around six-thirty a.m. and start to feel quasi-human by nine or so. That's my burnoff point. Although factors such as sleep, hydration, nutrition, stress, and exercise can influence my early morning pain, I know that by mid-morning I *should* begin to feel better.

Monitoring my burnoff point helps me gauge my progress. Burnoff is gradual, but the healthier and stronger I become, the earlier and more quickly burnoff arrives.

Another valuable tool to measure the effectiveness of a new exercise routine is to consider sleep patterns. Good sleep follows good exercise (and good nutrition, of course). After consistent workouts, ask yourself if you woke fewer times during the night. Did you toss and turn less? Sleep more deeply? Did you get to the REM stage of restorative sleep? Like burnoff, monitoring sleep patterns helps you analyze the merits of your workouts.

Look for these physical responses immediately after a workout. Do your muscles feel "spent," as if all the blood has drained away? Do you feel fatigued, possibly sweaty? If so, congratulations!

Being tired is good, but how long that feeling lasts tells you what you need to know. Do your muscles feel better in thirty minutes? An hour? Do your joints or muscles feel increased pain several hours after exercise? That's neither typical nor desirable.

Pay attention to these post-exercise factors, along with the following day's burnoff point. If you do, you'll be able to gauge the effectiveness of your exercise program. With a bit of practice, you'll be able to forecast your exercise success with a fair amount of accuracy.

WRAP IT UP

I do tai chi, aerobics (T-Tapp), weight machines at the gym, walking, rebounding on my trampoline, and whatever new, intriguing exercise I come across. These are my favorites; it's up to you to assemble your individualized collection. Vary the repertoire, and give any new exercise routine time to work. Be patient. It takes time for our bodies to adjust. Starting a new routine may involve muscles you haven't used in a while. Initial fatigue and some soreness are typical. Consider it an adjustment period.

If you're a "newbie," pay particular attention to posture as you exercise. If you're unsure about a pose or how to sit or stand on specific exercise equipment, ask a pro (preferably someone who understands the physiology of fibromyalgia). Even minor adjustments to your posture can help avoid injury.

Oh, and one more thing: remember to breathe! Pay attention to your breath. Is it regular? Even? Shallow? If you're not yet taking advantage of the circulation boost provided by a good, deep breath, it's time to start. Breathe deeply enough to expand your chest; a strong breath helps with stability as well as the cardiovascular system. The consistent breathing patterns found in exercises like yoga and tai chi also assist with relaxation.

This chapter covered moving the body through exercise. Breathing is a critical part of that as it oxygenates the muscles. Proper breathing also plays a role in stress-relieving activities as mentioned in the next chapter. When the body (via exercise) and the mind work in tandem, healing follows.

"You can have anything you want if you will give up the belief that you can't have it."

—Dr. Robert Anthony

Chapter 7

What'll it be—illness or wellness?

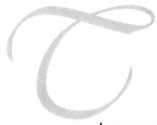he component of the restoration trio that runs the whole show is emotional wellness. How we *think* affects how we *feel*.

I've mentioned that action leads to improved health. Proper nutrition and exercise are all you need to whip you into shape, right?

Wrong. Something's missing.

The MIND is where *plan* and *action* intersect. Wellness doesn't "come and knock on our door" like nosey Mr. Roper from the seventies sitcom, *Three's Company*. Wellness must be sought out, locked into the crosshairs. Luckily for us, the mind is perfectly suited for crosshair focus.

Eating like a yogi and exercising like an Olympian is great; but, without a mental strategy, you're critically handicapped. Changes in diet and exercise alone won't fix all ills. Figuring out *how* you think about your health is primary.

Emotional wellness is so vital to the restoration trio, that I placed it last—like Santa Claus in the Macy's Thanksgiving Day parade. Do you *think* you can rebuild wellness? Do you *think* there are solutions to your health problems?

Even if you said no, you're not off the hook. I'm not saying you can simply think your way to wellness (although there's a kernel of truth in that concept), but, every journey has a beginning. *Better health begins with the conviction to seek it.* If you're heck-bent on finding an answer, you eventually will. Tenacity pays off.

Answer two questions. First, do you truly want to seek wellness? Second, are you open-minded enough to recognize the answers you find? Finding answers means time spent in self-discovery. The following sections of this chapter will help pave the way.

STRESS FOR SUCCESS

Stress, as destructive as toxic waste, has the capacity to compromise health at the cellular level. Stress negatively affects the immune and digestive systems, cognitive abilities, even physical attributes, such as skin, hair, and nails.

Stress alters moods. It's not fun being around "stressed out" people. There are those who spread cheer and those who spread the emotional equivalent of the bubonic plague. That's emotional toxicity.

Here's a brief physiology lesson. Stress causes the sympathetic nervous system to become agitated (for us fibrofolk, that's a real pain). Stress-relieving activities activate the parasympathetic nervous system, resulting in physical benefits such as muscle relaxation and mental clarity.

Activities that relieve stress, therefore, have wide-reaching effects.

The following modalities are known to counteract stress. These overviews are far from comprehensive. Seek more information on any or all to which you feel drawn.

- Prayer
- Meditation
- MTT (Meridian Tapping Technique)
- Journaling
- Imagery
- Massage
- Humor

Prayer and meditation are probably the two most familiar stress-busters and MTT possibly the least familiar. Journaling, imagery, massage, and humor are all great de-stressors. Try them all!

These tools, along with diet and exercise, may provide everything needed to complete your wellness plan.

PRAYER

Prayer is personal, a topic to address with sensitivity and respect. For some, it's a reverent act done with ceremony. For others, it's simply talking to God as a personal BFF (best friend forever).

We each pray in different ways. Prayers can be free-flowing, formulaic, consistent, sporadic, ongoing, concise. Ultimately, prayer helps us develop a personal relationship with our Maker. It's good to know the universe is bigger than just us. That spiritual connection gives us a sense of belonging, a sense of identity.

If you think of prayer as one-way conversation, you're missing out on half the benefits. Even while you're talking (praying), you're enjoying physiological as well as spiritual payoffs. Confession of the soul brings comfort. Sharing grief, pain, or worries can reduce anxiety, lower blood pressure, increase blood flow, boost the immune system, and induce mood-enhancing benefits.

Prayer is one of the simplest modalities for stress management. What's easier than talking? No complicated skills necessary. If you're unsure or uncomfortable with any aspect of prayer, ask God for help. Talk out your concerns and worries. Give thanks for your joys. The more you converse, the more comfortable you'll feel.

Pray for help, guidance, understanding, or forgiveness, and include others in your petitions. Talk about anything and everything. A prayer journal is a good way to remember your prayers. Periodically, flip back to prior pages in your journal to see how your prayers have been answered. *Answers aren't always as we expect.*

The act of forgiveness is a powerful healing tool — for both the forgiver and the forgivee. Holding a grudge can make you physically sick. Harboring anger, resentment, or bitterness towards another is a lonely and pointless pursuit. Forgiveness may help the one you're forgiving; but ultimately, the greatest benefit is yours.

Think you're too busy to pray? We all have days filled with responsibilities and unfinished tasks. Pray anytime you're alone: on a walk, in the kitchen, car, gym, grocery store, office. When you're alone with your thoughts, you're never really alone.

Make prayer a daily habit, but don't worry. God is always tuned in, even when we're not.

MEDITATION

Meditation is a paradox; simply complex. It's easier to talk than to listen, and, for this reason, many people (including me) find it easier to pray than to meditate. It takes time to develop a meditative skill, but the benefits are vastly rewarding. Meditation is relaxing, of course, but that's just a start. Reduced blood pressure, anxiety, and pain are desirable side effects.

I once heard some people say meditation is for lazy people, all that "sitting still." They couldn't be more wrong. Relaxation takes action. It's *choosing* to care for yourself enough to recharge your batteries. Yes, meditation is about inaction, but it's the purposeful aspect of it that's beneficial.

Meditation is called an art for a reason. Some grasp the nuances faster than others, but persistence pays. No one begins their meditative journey as a pro. Find your own comfort level. Remember the adage: Anything worth doing well takes practice.

Novice or pro, be kind to yourself. The mind wanders; we're not a society comfortable with stillness. It's not as important what you think as how you think. Do your best to eliminate negative or pointless emotions such as guilt and shame. Negative thinking is an unwelcome but common mental intruder. Don't get too wrapped up with trying to plan what to think about. Let your thoughts come and go of their own accord.

Meditation helps to corral and sort out counterproductive thoughts. It provides clarity. You might choose to read up on meditation methods, and select some soothing nature sounds or relaxation CDs.

Enlist all of your senses, and don't forget your nose. Your sense of smell can be a powerful part of the meditation experience. The olfactory sense links directly to the brain, and your memory can evoke an immediate response. Use your favorite scented flowers, candles, or soothing, natural, essential oils.

Meditation has proven benefits. Hospitals use meditation to help surgery patients. Improvements in post-surgery healing takes place when patients are calm, relaxed, and have a positive outlook. How does this relate to you? Amid kids' soccer games, work, grocery store runs, and volunteer meetings, you may wonder when, exactly, the relaxation will start.

Stress is the problem, and relieving stress is the answer.

One definition of stress is this: feeling the demands placed on you are greater than your ability to deal with them. Sound familiar? It's time to take action by choosing inaction. Slow down. Get focused. Everyone complains about stress, but how many people actively do something to relieve it?

Here's where you can become proactive. Invest time in relaxation (meditation and prayer) and *make it a priority*. You'll experience benefits that far exceed your expectations.

Be forewarned. Meditation can remove you, mentally, from the concepts of time and space. So, if you hear, "Have you lost your mind?"

The answer is, "You noticed? Thanks!"

MTT (Meridian Tapping Technique)

While this may be one of the oddest-looking activities you've ever seen, MTT boasts an impressive success rate. Widely known as a powerful cognitive healing tool (though one of the most underused), it's free. Did you catch that? FREE.

MTT combines Eastern medicine's healing practices, such as acupuncture, with the mental health treatments of Western medicine. Even better, it's a shortcut to both.

Simply put, MTT is the practice of tapping on the body while talking or thinking of problem issues. Most tapping points are strategically located along acupressure energy meridians on the upper body and hands.

MTT can be used to help resolve *any* issue, emotional or physical. It can help with stress reduction, pain management, goal-setting, eating habits, or to help improve physical performance in sports.

There are as many varieties of MTT methods as there are practitioners, and access is often free and abundant. Search online and you'll find videos; varieties of people performing MTT on a myriad of phobias and problems.

The widespread options of MTT are plentiful. It's easiest to begin at the Emotional Freedom Technique (EFT®) website[18] from founder, Gary Craig. You'll find a free, downloadable manual and plenty of information. It's simple to learn; don't fret about details. Familiarize yourself with the technique, get the gist, and then look for practical examples. Surf video websites such as http://www.youtube.com/ and find the techniques and the practitioners you

---

18.   http://www.emofree.com/ [accessed 02/02/10]

find appealing. Books and DVDs such as *Try It On Everything*[19] may prove helpful.

Be patient if the "woo hoo" lingo of some practitioners turns you off. Remember, you're only watching and learning until you get the hang of it. Find practitioners who seem in line with your needs and ignore the rest. Most important are their words and the sound of their voices. Many speak in peaceful tones, but some are less-than soothing. Listen for voices that make you feel relaxed and comfortable. Surf, click, and listen.

Weight loss and behavior modification guru Paul McKenna[20] demonstrates a hybrid version of tapping methods on his videos. To me, his voice is charismatic enough to sell popsicles to Eskimos.

You can also find qualified practitioners in your area who instruct MTT in person. Learning MTT over the phone is also common. These are "fee-based" services but may be worth every penny. Don't be afraid to ask for references. Ask questions to ensure a good fit for both of you. I've found that MTT newbies tend to focus on minutia. Don't sweat the details. Here are answers to common newbie questions: Tap with either hand or both. Tap on either side of your body, or tap on one side and then move to the other. Use the tips of your fingers or whatever feels comfortable. You don't need to count the number of taps. Don't worry if you don't know what to say; you'll find your own dialogue with practice.

MTT is a surprisingly forgiving technique. Just do it; you can't go wrong.

People resistant to new things can get creative with their objections. Threatened by the simplicity of MTT, some try to make it more difficult than it is.

"My nails are too long," (then, don't use your nails; use the pads of your fingertips).
"My finger hurts," (so don't use that finger or don't tap so hard).
"I get dizzy when I close my eyes," (so don't close your eyes).
"I can't concentrate if I'm standing," (so sit).
"I don't know what to say," (so say what someone else says until

---

19.   http://www.thetappingsolution.com/index2.php/ [accessed 01/31/10]
20.   http://www.mckenna.com/ [accessed 01/10/10]

your own dialogue feels natural).

"I can't talk and tap at the same time," (so sorry, can't help you there).

As with anything new, be kind to yourself. Be persistent. Keep an open mind. Soon, you'll be proficient on your own. You'll sync your own words with your issues. That's the epitome of individualized healing.

I often hear questions such as, "I wonder if MTT works on migraines, insomnia, phobias, food cravings, memory issues, or to improve my golf swing, etc.?" The answer is, "yes."

Instead of saying, "I wonder if MTT works," say "MTT works wonders!"

JOURNALING

Simply putting your troubles into words can relieve stress. Journaling is effective, and writing out your worries is a good place to start. It's not a stress-relieving technique available only to creative souls. If you can write, you can journal.

Words are powerful.

Words can express and heal.

Details matter. First, choose a pen that feels good to you. Choose a journal in your favorite color or material. Don't overlook the importance of your writing instruments; they reflect your personality. Besides, they'll be with you through thick and thin.

Begin by writing about goals or plans. Who are you today? Who do you want to be tomorrow? Keep it simple. In journaling, honesty is valued above eloquence. Be sure to sign your goals list or life plan. Your signature seals your commitment to take action.

What's the best time to write? At bedtime, you can encapsulate your day. Jot down your blessings and people for whom you're thankful. Maybe morning is more your style. Start your day with a short paragraph of free thought. Try your hand at poetry or prose. Write a few words on each line and, no, they don't have to rhyme.

Your journal is yours alone. Write to suit yourself; no judgment allowed. That goes for everyone — especially you.

Once you start, you may find you've more to say than you thought possible. Writing unlocks the subconscious, giving you access to tucked-away thoughts and feelings. Don't over-analyze what you write. If something you write shocks or concerns you, keep writing. The more you write, the more you'll learn about yourself.

That's the essence of healing. Learning about yourself allows you to pinpoint beneficial and not-so-beneficial thoughts and behaviors. Are your thoughts self-critical? Worrisome? Judgmental? Journaling can help determine the cause of negative thinking. Rooting out the cause puts healing in motion.

Through journaling, a "word picture" of you may develop. Your personality might come into sharper focus. Try on a new wardrobe of words. Words can be telling, loving, interesting, and often surprising. Words that you feel are not "you" (such as creative, free-thinking, peace-filled) may become the best fit of all.

IMAGERY

Using mental images as a stress-relieving tool is nothing new. Imagery has been used in therapeutic environments for centuries. Mental images have a physiological affect on the body. In fact, the body is unable to discern the difference between real experiences and those that are vividly imagined. Some imagery techniques use a voice (recorded or live) to mentally take you to a place of relaxation. Unlike prayer and meditation, imagery has a destination or goal — physical and mental relaxation. Imagery can take you to your "happy place."

Imagery can be done with or without a guide and is especially helpful in times of conflict. In meetings, waiting rooms, or even a noisy gym, taking a mental trip to my happy place reaps physical rewards such as stabilized heart rate and reduced anxiety. I've developed my own customized version of imagery. Find a version (or vision!) that works for you.

I love Hawaii. That's not a tough sell. I once mentioned to a fellow traveler that, although I visit often, I still love the sights, sounds, and scents of Waikiki. He looked shocked. Oahu is the megalopolis of Hawaii and Waikiki the epicenter: far-too-developed in the opinion of many tourists.

We'd seen the same city, but through different experiences. I'm a history buff. While others don swimwear and head toward the surf, I find museums, libraries, national landmarks. I'm probably the only tourist who's spent entire days at the Hawaiian National Archives.

From my hotel's fifth floor balcony, I overlook Kalakaua Avenue, facing the majestic Moana Surfrider Hotel. I know there's a confluence of traffic and tourists below, but, instead, I see the column-lined porte-cochère of the Surfrider. I see it, in my mind's -eye, as it stood a century ago. I feel the ocean breezes, listen to the cooing of tiny Hawaiian doves. I hear the low moan of a giant ocean liner's air horn and imagine restless passengers waiting to disembark. I sense their eagerness for adventure.

I step into prior eras of Hawaiian life as easily as into capris and flip flops.

"The greatest discovery of my generation is that a human being can alter his life by altering his attitudes of mind."

—William James

This is where I go, mentally, when I feel squeezed by the "real world." A few moments of this imagery, and I'm able to let go of tensions and worries. This respite supplies me with renewed energy to face my next challenge.

Imagery can be customized to suit your needs. Experiment with imagery CDs or library books. Hawaii does it for me, but where is your happy place? A vacation memory? A childhood hideout? Thoughts of your favorite park, shore, library, place of worship, or even shopping mall can bring a sense of wholeness and peace. To each his own.

Whatever it is, simply thinking about it can make puddles of stress evaporate. Or maybe it's not a place at all? Some people experience "happy hormones" (endorphins) when gardening, running, bicycling, skiing, or surfing. Find an activity that soothes your worried soul. Think of times when you've felt calm and relaxed. Did the physical location and experience leave its mark on you or was it the activity? Either way, that's your happy place.

What is it about your special place that makes you happy? Examine your surroundings. What do you see, hear, taste, smell, and feel? Imbue those thoughts with color and heightened sensations to maximize the relaxation benefits. When you think of your happy place, turn up the colors as if adjusting your TV or computer monitor. Envision the blues brighter, the greens deeper. Include feelings such as comfort, safety, and gratitude. Make your mental picture as vivid as possible. Then visit your custom-made happy place any time you wish — no inoculations or passport required.

MASSAGE

If you think massage is not a valuable stress-relieving tool, I'd wager you've never had one. A good massage soothes you physically and mentally. In fact, if insurance companies were truly interested in preventative medicine, regular massage would be covered under most plans.

A massage doesn't simply feel good. Therapeutic massage can create chemical changes within the body to alleviate pain. Massage can reduce substance P (a protein found in the brain related to pain) and thereby help chronically ill people, including those with fibromyalgia, arthritis conditions, migraines, and back troubles. Boosted immune systems, reduced stress, and lowered blood pressure are additional benefits of massage.

Like finding the right fitness trainer, it may take time to ferret out the perfect massage therapist. Interview them as you would any other trained professional. Discuss your goals and symptoms. Talk about the results you expect, and define what types of touch you prefer. If you don't feel understood, go elsewhere. It's counterproductive to find yourself the day afterward sore enough to mitigate the benefits.

But *do* keep looking for the right massage therapist. It's worth the investment. The right therapist is out there waiting to bring you that special healing touch. This is one instance where — if you seek, you will unwind.

HUMOR

Chronic illness helps you to become decisive. You might plan on three errands, but your body decides one and a half will do. Like arguing with your mother, arguing with your body is rarely fruitful.

Having a sense of humor about your chronic illness is more important than all the prior healing treatments put together. I don't take myself as seriously as I did in the past and have learned to laugh at my condition — and at myself.

I wasn't particularly graceful to begin with, but fibromyalgia has taught me to execute pratfalls and fumbles like a comedic pro. No, I haven't done a swan dive over my ottoman, Dick Van Dyke-style, but I frequently stumble on mine. If I don't laugh with the others, well then, that would be sad, wouldn't it?

Denial is another option. I could pretend my poor dexterity doesn't exist, or that I *plan* to trip over the threshold to the video store — every single time. But that wouldn't honor the real me. I am someone who doesn't always know what my extremities are doing, and I've got the scarred knees to prove it.

A sense of humor about where we find ourselves keeps us grounded. It also helps us prioritize (i.e., pain to the background, enjoyable activity to the foreground). Have you ever gone to a funny movie with a headache and forgotten the pain? What about giggling at lunch with good friends? Laughter is balm for any wound.

Laughing is beneficial in other ways, too. It can increase your body's ability to fight infection, create a sense of wellness, and, best of all, it needs no translation. Laughter speaks in every tongue.

If you can't laugh about finding your car keys in the cupboard next to the soup bowls, another option is to cry. Cognitive dysfunction is often part of chronic illness, and pretending won't make the incidences go away. Accept them for what they are.

No, pain can't be ignored, and, no, it isn't funny. But life sure is. Funny things can and do still happen, even after a chronic illness diagnosis. This fact remains: Laughter is not only fun, it's therapeutic.

OUR CHOICES MAKE ALL THE DIFFERENCE

Sylvia was referred to me out of desperation. I was told she'd "tried everything" to relieve her symptoms. In our first phone conversation, she blurted out a litany of prescription medications she took, including dosages down to the milligram. She listed what medicated topical creams she applied, along with where and when. She seamlessly detailed her experiences with physical therapy, x-rays, MRIs, and brain scans. She identified what parts of her body hurt the day before and what parts were in pain at the moment. She told me what her husband thought of her health problems and what her children told her to do. I heard her co-workers' opinions as well as her mother's. (I heard about Sylvia's cat, Charlie, and expected to hear what he thought of her illness.) Sylvia was a potential candidate for the fast-talkers recovery group, On and On and On-Anon.

My conversation with Sylvia is not unusual among those with chronic illness. I listen and wedge in comments when able.

Sick people need to vent.

They need to share ideas, concerns, and worries. The Sylvias of this world are overwhelmed, and rightly so. Illness is the focus of their lives. Thoughts, both conscious and subconscious, are all about being sick. A chronically ill "Sylvia" manages her illness as a CEO manages a corporation.

I'm not making light of the situation; I was there once, too. I remember the frustrations and worries about each new pain, new doctor, new medication. I now have the clarity that's borne of experience. I recognize a misalignment of focus in Sylvia.

What would happen if Sylvia focused as much attention on wellness as on illness?

I suggested to Sylvia that she try stress-relieving activities. I encouraged her to find tai chi or yoga classes in her neighborhood. I offered ideas on how to incorporate prayer and meditation into her busy life. Did she listen? Truthfully, I sensed her mind spun too fast to hear me, but at least I planted the seeds.

I make the same suggestion here. It probably sounds ridiculous to try tai chi if your pain level is so high you can barely get out of bed. Struggling to a yoga class full of strangers may be the last thing you feel like doing, but at least consider it. Think about it, and let that thought run through your mind often. Imagine caring for your body, nurturing it. Think of what you *can* do rather than what you cannot. We all have options. Thinking about them can turn the tide of our focus.

What happens if you think about making changes to your daily routine? Start by beginning to think of wellness as a possibility. That "beginning place" becomes the focus.

I often hear, "I don't have time," when I mention stress-relieving methods. The obvious answer is that your body will *make* time for you. People, like Sylvia, who mentally run in circles, get nowhere. Their mental misalignment adds to their physical suffering.

The body does what it needs to get attention.

Are you listening to your body's messages? It's time to shift your focus. Live in the "beginning place," and soon your choices will reflect your thoughts. It's a matter of focus and, it's up to you.

THE ROAD TO CHIRO

Years ago, my chiropractor's response to my fibromyalgia diagnosis was, "You're not buying that, are you? We all have morning aches and pains." She acted as if I'd sought my diagnosis for self-serving purposes.

I felt crushed. She didn't understand fibromyalgia at all. We'd had a long-term relationship, and I thought she knew me. I didn't want attention — I wanted answers!

Time for a new chiropractor.

Chiropractors are typically outside-the-box thinkers. Looking at the body as a whole instead of the sum of its parts, they seek systemic solutions. Their specialties vary widely, so I sought the right one for me.

I researched local practitioners, asking about their fibromyalgia know-how. Dr. DoGood's response perplexed me. He expressed familiarity with fibromyalgia, but sounded ambivalent about treating it. How odd. In my experience, practitioners either know nothing (and hope you go away), or claim to know everything (and want you to begin *their* treatments ASAP).

Piqued, I made an appointment. As a sports chiropractor, he listened while I told him my frustrations with the limitations fibromyalgia put on my exercise routines. He sighed deeply and looked relieved.

Then Dr. DoGood said something I've often retold. "From my experience, there are two types of fibromyalgia patients: those who want to get better and those who don't. You obviously want to get better, and I'm very happy to meet you."

I've thought a lot about that comment over the years. It's sad, but profound. I don't think Dr. DoGood's comment is completely accurate, but I understand his point. Chronically ill people often *do* fall into one of two camps. Some actively seek solutions while others succumb to hopelessness.

I have a theory about why some give up hope of getting better. First, the insidious nature of chronic illness wears down even the hardiest people. Add to that, repeated dismissals from the medical community, and the silent resignation (and sometimes resentment) of family and friends. Who wouldn't feel isolated, angry, and defeated?

At this point, a fork appears in the road. Some seek solutions, and others accept their diagnosis as if it's a stagnant, unyielding entity.

> *"The richness of the human experience would lose something of rewarding joy if there were no limitations to overcome."*
>
> —Helen Keller

My theory on which fork people take depends on one major factor: time. How long did they search for answers? How many doctors and health professionals slammed doors in their faces? How prolonged were their "waffled" and "pancaked" stages? (Remember Chapter Four?)

Other factors include individual personality traits, the support (or non-support) of family and friends, and work/financial pressures. In general, the longer a person suffers in silence or is forced to walk the health maze alone, the more a person begins to identify with his or her condition. That's the kicker. For some, the word fibromyalgia becomes *who* they are — not *what* they have. They *are* fibromyalgia (or chronic fatigue, rheumatoid arthritis, lupus, Crohn's disease, Epstein-barr, diabetes, cancer, etc.). They make statements such as, "I'm not well today because of *my* chronic fatigue," sounding as if they own or have purchased the condition.

They wear the cloak of their illness everywhere. They assume its identity and no longer exist outside that definition. Strangely, that identity provides a level of comfort, or safety. Their *I am* statements may sound like this: "I am disabled. I am different. I am unable to work/play. I am set apart. I am broken. I am special."

That "specialness" provides justification for not participating. But it's not as simple as skipping a high school gym class; it's skipping out *on life.*

People who "become" their illness cannot see any other self, cannot see themselves as anything other than disabled. In fact, to take away that disability (suggesting wellness as an option) may be perceived as threatening. Many chronically ill people throw up roadblocks at any chance for improvement or recovery. They aren't willing to try treatment options that take action or personal investment, because it's too risky. What if the treatments didn't work? Or what if they became well and discovered they were not who they thought they were? *Who* would they be instead?

Fibromyalgia (or any other chronic illness) is merely *one aspect* of self.

I'd like to tweak Dr. DoGood's theory a bit. I believe sick people really do want to get better; they just *don't know how.*

Rebuilding wellness begins when the label of chronic illness is put in its place; when it becomes simply one descriptor. Patients *can* achieve wellness through action and tenacity. I'm sure the observant Dr. DoGood would concur.

YOU'RE NOT THE BOSS OF ME!

In a skit at my church, one friend played an agitated, sick woman in an emergency room. With dramatic flair, she moaned, groaned, and swayed. She was convincing. Curious, I asked her, afterward, how she felt.

"Funny you ask," she said. "I made myself so sick I thought I'd throw up! I'll have to tone it down next time; my stomach is still in knots."

She demonstrated the powerful connection between mind and body. You *can* make yourself feel sick. Doesn't it stand to reason you can also make yourself feel *well?*

Your mind is the *primary* tool in your health arsenal. Do you *think* you'll get better? Do you *think* you deserve good health? Do you *think* you'll be successful in restoring your health? (HINT: The answer to all of the above is, YES.)

Your thoughts lead you, but to where? I have dear friends who are each activists for health, parenting, or political issues. They could be perceived as bossy. Their faces light up as they "fight the good fight" for their beliefs. Their actions demonstrate a visceral connection to their cause; their dedication is admirable.

It may seem an odd coincidence, but many of these same friends suffer from physical ills. Some deal with migraines, IBS, diabetes, and cancer. Is there a connection?

Passionate people tend to prioritize their lives using their cause as the ultimate litmus test. If an activity furthers that cause, it tops their to-do list. If not, it may not make honorable mention. Their health needs fall pitifully low on their list of priorities.

The brain is adept at setting priorities and defining goals. When you focus on a balanced lifestyle, you'll see a corresponding shift in priorities. However, if you don't *decide* to care for your health, decisions will be made for you.

Feed your brain the information it needs to map out a healing plan. Let your mind focus on healing thoughts, and you'll experience a shift in priorities. In this instance, being bossy is a good thing.

I AM READY, WILLING, AND ABLE

What you think about your health allows you to be right — every time. Do you think a diet will work? No? Then, you're right. Think exercise is too hard to fit into your daily routine? Right again!

Some say the two most powerful words in the English language are *I am*. Whatever follows proves true. Think about it. Do you say things like, *I am never on time*, or *I am so disorganized*? If so, odds are you're habitually tardy or have a cluttered desk.

What other *I am* statements do you make? *I am in pain. I am unheard. I am always sick. I am handicapped. I am unable to manage my eating habits.* Do these words or phrases truly describe you? Are they the words you *want* to describe you?

Many of us struggle between what we want and what we feel we deserve. The paradox is that people who are unhappy about where they are can't be "present" anywhere else.

When thoughts are at odds with goals, forward motion is impossible. Make your mind work *for* you instead of *against* you. By implementing healing modalities to clear away wellness roadblocks, your goals will sharpen into focus. You can reframe your *I am* statements, keeping your new goals in mind. Choose powerful, positive, and healing thoughts.

Make up your mind *now* to focus on a healthier future. The wellness brass ring is right there — within your grasp.

ATTRACTION IS AS ATTRACTION DOES

I try to choose activities that revitalize rather than demobilize me. I've learned from past mistakes. I used to overdo the joining, volunteering, and meeting thing. Still, I felt I wasn't doing enough. I addressed Christmas cards in council sessions and crocheted afghans during choir practice. It's entirely possible that those organizations don't miss me much.

Of course, my problem wasn't in doing enough; it was my inability to prioritize my activities. Each task I chose shortchanged another. I failed at being truly present anywhere.

That was my mental game. I cared for my basic physical needs, ignoring my emotional ones.

On the path to healing, the mind is our greatest ally and our greatest adversary. So, how do we reconcile spinning thoughts and find balance?

The answer depends on your personality. Some people need physical activity to sort out emotional issues. Repetitive motion such as knitting, gardening, or riding a cruiser bike can be helpful. For others, physical intensity provides a mental solution. They benefit from activities such as kickboxing, aerobics, or tennis.

Others may find that stillness silences the mental chatter. Being truly present, particularly in nature, can sharpen ideas into focus.

Physical activities can relieve stress in a tangible way. Keep an open mind as you try new things. Early attempts may seem futile or clumsy, but, when you get the hang of it, you'll begin to relish a feeling of emotional calm. It may even become as addictive as the adrenaline rush you formerly chased.

There's currently a lot of media attention about emotional calm and attracting good things. It's a popular topic, but the foundations of attraction are older than the printed word. Not much has changed in thousands of years. Prayer and meditation are the same today as ever. When you spend more time in self-discovery than worrying about the business of others, emotional balance is your reward.

People who are balanced and calm naturally attract balanced and calm solutions to their problems.

Notice I didn't say they have no problems. Balanced people have problems just like everyone else. The difference is in how they deal with those problems. They don't react out of fear or anxiety. Instead, their reactions are typically rational, reasonable, and well-thought-out.

Dealing with racing thoughts is the first step to de-stressing. It's more than taking a break. When you're able to calm your mind, you remove yourself from the stressful situation. That respite and detachment gives you the clarity to make better decisions and seek better solutions. You'll gain a different view of your concerns, and that fresh focus allows you to recognize opportunities otherwise missed.

WHADDAYA LOOKIN' FOR?

I have friends who always talk about buying a home. One day I asked to hear what steps they'd taken. Had they consulted a Realtor or checked any real estate websites? No. Had they driven around desirable neighborhoods on Sundays or saved for a down payment? No, and not at all.

They must believe their dream home will plop down from the sky, like Dorothy's house into Munchkinland. Fact is, if they truly wanted a home, their actions would match their words.

Many of us are walking contradictions. We say we want magazine articles on healthy living, yet issues featuring decadent desserts on the covers fly off the shelves. Maybe your behavior is contradictory, too. Do you *really* want good health? What actions have you taken? You don't have to re-vamp every aspect of your life, but you do have to start somewhere.

Say what you mean and mean what you say. If you want good health, what habits are you willing to change to achieve it?

This is where many people jump to the opposite extreme. I hear, "I could never be a health nut!" Well, neither could I. There's a *big* difference between inaction and fanaticism. Where we fit on the spectrum of "health nut" is only relative to someone else's ideas.

I invite you to check it out for yourself. The world of healthy living is a safe and comfortable place to be; I promise.

THE PEACH PARADIGM

I want to give credit where credit is due. I often discuss my health analogies with my husband. Writing is a solitary pursuit, which makes writers rather poor company when we're working. And the select few who do hang around me bear the brunt of comments such as, "Hey! Listen to what psyllium seed husks do to the digestive tract!"

One day while researching, I talked about how latent emotional issues can turn into physical symptoms. My practical spouse made a comment that became the basis for the following analogy. I have to admit, it's a peach.

Let's say you have an unresolved issue. We'll assume that somewhere in your past, you were emotionally wounded. To illustrate, a peach represents that emotional wound.

You know the peach exists, but you don't want to see it or think about it. You put the peach in a cupboard and slam the door. Problem solved.

Eventually, you smell something strange. You open the cupboard. The peach is moldy, shriveled; the stink is nauseating. You go to a professional for advice. He suggests a trip to the hardware store to purchase a sticky-backed air freshener. That'll fix it!

The peach still stinks. Another professional suggests that the discolored wood in the cupboard is contributing to the smell. Special cleaning wipes are needed. You scrub the cupboard inside and out — all around that gnarly, decrepit peach. You're exhausted, but at least it's been taken care of.

Until … you enter your kitchen and smell rancid fruit, scented air freshener, *and* bleach.

You open the cupboard door; a black, misshapen lump stares back at you. The peach. The cupboard is stained and doesn't look like the others. You get out a brush and roller to give it a quick once-over, but flies stick to the wet paint. You consult with yet another professional and learn you need a pest control expert.

You've spent time and money on professionals, fragrances,

cleaners, paint, and an exterminator. You're exhausted, spent in more ways than one.

One last time, you seek the advice of a professional. You find a "big picture" person who looks at the health of your kitchen as a whole. She says the word "peach" and you bristle with indignation. How dare she bring *that* up?

She gently points out that the other problems will always exist as long as the peach exists. In fact, they'll multiply. Perhaps it's time to deal with the peach?

In this illustration, are the smells, stained cupboard, and flies real? It's important to note that they're as real as the symptoms we experience with our illnesses.

Problems persist as long as unresolved issues (peaches) continue to negatively affect us. Unresolved issues may not be *the* problem, but it's a place to start.

Emotional wounds, given time, turn into physical ones. And, they need as much attention.

Emotional wounds may stem from events done either to or by us. Resentment has no positive outcome. Like bat guano in our mental caves, resentment builds, serving no purpose other than to obscure our view of reality. While we can't rewrite history, we can choose how we wish to view it.

Ask yourself, "Who would I be if I no longer carried this burden? What positive thoughts would fill the gaps left by the absence of regret, pain, anger, or resentment?"

Dealing with core problems in a healthy way alleviates mental and physical symptoms. Enlist the wisdom of a counselor if you have difficulty identifying core issues. Focusing on what's "hidden" in your cupboards today may save you from major kitchen remodelling tomorrow. Clearing old issues may be "the pits," but isn't that the true nature of a peach?

THE PAIN NETWORK

In my childhood home, our only TV had a dial, no remote control, three channels, and a nebulous UHF notch to tune in snowy programs. TV reception was more miss than hit.

I now understand transmissions may be sent by the station,

but a TV is only as good as its ability to receive those signals. The receiver is the gatekeeper.

Receivers, in general, can be programmed to accept desired transmissions and ignore the undesirable. Only *invited* transmissions are received.

This "invitation only" concept applies to pain receivers, too. We're receptive to some messages, energies, and intentions and not others. What do we choose to receive?

I thought about this once after going to a movie. A tiny irritant fell into my eye just as the movie started. It's amazing how something so tiny can cause such intense pain. I didn't want to miss the opening scenes and wondered what to do.

Thankfully, minor eye irritations usually resolve themselves. The body naturally increases moisture and lubrication in the troubled eye. The resolution occurs regardless of your focus.

> "*All truths are easy to understand once they are discovered; the point is to discover them.*"
>
> —Galileo

That's exactly what happened. I became interested in the movie, forgot about the irritant, and the pain "went away." In other words, I changed the channel of my focus; my pain went from foreground transmission to background. It was no longer invited.

Pain transmissions occur whether we focus on them or not. That ability to shift focus from pain is one of the principles of the Lamaze childbirth technique. Labor pains are managed by shifting our focus to visual and breathing cues.

To manage chronic pain, we do have a choice about what kind of "receivers" we wish to be. We don't have to tune in to the All Pain Network where it's all pain, all the time.

It's up to us. We're in charge of the remote control; we have the power to change the channel.

LIVE IN THE SKIN

A serious actor might do a character study and "live in the skin" of his character. The persona becomes so real, the actor doesn't feel as if he's acting.

Acting isn't only for those in Hollywood. You can choose to "act" as a healthy person; take a starring role as someone healthy, fit, and able-bodied. How would it feel to live in the skin of someone with healthy muscles and a pain-free spine? How would she treat her body? Is a healthy body worthy of care and respect?

Give it a try. See how it feels to think and live as a healthy person. It starts with acting, but familiarity settles in. When you think, feel, and treat yourself as a healthy person, it's no longer make-believe. You'll find that the health and confidence you attain is deeper than the skin you're in.

FOCUS POCUS

Thoughts are powerful. They drive our actions. The question is: How do we make practical use of this knowledge?

Be mindful. Become aware of your focus. What thoughts course wildly through your brain? What concerns and worst-case scenarios do you mentally replay? What thoughts are keeping you stuck in the past? Do you worry about family, finances, work, diet, or exercise?

We nurture the things we want to grow: our children, businesses, relationships. Can we also nurture and grow traits or characteristics? That's a matter of focus. Some of us focus on frenzied thoughts and then seem surprised by a flourishing "crop of crazy."

What we think about most is the true object of our focus. That's what we nurture, what we want to grow. If we worry about failing in business, that's what we'll achieve. If we worry about our declining health, we'll see that to fruition.

Where we choose to focus is the problem, and changing that focus is the solution. For example, let's say your focus is on a negative body image. You obsess over your perceived shortcomings and exaggerate every bump, bulge, and bounce. Your distorted ideas affect other aspects of your life. If you consistently think negative thoughts about your body, then no diet or exercise program can succeed. Your body cannot change.

You are as you believe.

It's up to you to change the channel of your thoughts to a healthier station. Think about areas in your life you'd like to change. List

your preferred focus items as goals and put them into action.
Here's an example of how this works:

Jane's Personal Goals
1. Get healthy.
2. Get a promotion.
3. Get the kids to focus more on family than on their computers.
4. Get organized. Find the book borrowed from John and return it.

To achieve these goals, Jane keeps her list handy and refers to it often. She also handwrites copies for her bathroom mirror, fridge, desk, and planner. Through repetition, Jane learns to replace negative thoughts with positive ones.

Feeling hopeful, she sets her plans into motion.

ITEM ONE. *Taking Better Care of Jane*
- Jane learns more about nutrition.
- She experiments with healthier recipes.
- She takes walks with the family after dinner.
- Encouraged, she begins an exercise program before work.
- She learns small changes provide big results.

ITEM TWO. *Getting Jane a Promotion*
- She looks into job training opportunities in her community.
- She volunteers to lead the next big project at the office.
- Using her new skills to spiff up her resumé, she seeks a job change and makes that promotion happen.

ITEM THREE. *Improving Jane's Family Communication*
- After work, Jane enlists her children to help with meal preparation.

- She engages her family in communication-enhancing activities such as Game Night, regular dinners at the table, and family-friendly outings.

ITEM FOUR. *Find John's Book and Return It*
- Spurred by her new-found energy, Jane clears clutter in her home and organizes her den. She finds the elusive book under her favorite reading chair and returns it to John.
- She proves there's merit to writing down all goals — big and small.

In the above scenario, you can see the importance of defining goals. What works for Jane can work for you. It's also important to share your goals with others. Sharing provides accountability and support. Sharing your goals tells others that, "These are the desires of my heart." Those who care for you support you. (Remember to dismiss comments and actions that feel unsupportive. *You* get to decide which to keep and which to toss.)

If this example were a Hollywood screenplay, Jane would transform from frumpy housewife to waif-sized corporate mogul. Before THE END floats across the screen, she'd sign a two-book deal for her titles, *See Jane Run* and *Family Dynamics: Chat Room to Dining Room.*

Hollywood, however, isn't real life. Jane's struggles may not merit a Lifetime movie of the week, but they're important, nonetheless. Jane made positive changes, and they all began with one step. She dreamed of a positive future and then planned for a positive future. She wrote down a goals list. No genie, no fairy godmother, no magic potion. Jane took action.

You can take action, too. Redirecting your thoughts isn't a quick fix, but it becomes easier with practice. Be patient. Write your own script. As with any good plot, it takes time to develop.

Give yourself permission to change your focus.

When Jane focused on a positive future, she replaced unhealthy thoughts with healthy ones. When it comes to examples, see Jane; follow Jane; run with Jane.

BUCKLE UP AND HAVE A SAFE FIGHT-OR-FLIGHT

Imagine your house is ablaze. You sprint between the inferno and your car, trying to salvage family heirlooms. Your mind races; your muscles strain.

During this crisis, would you stop to balance your checkbook? What about folding and putting away that last load of laundry? That's silly. Clean socks are not at the top of anyone's priority list during a crisis.

Your body's basic functions have a list of priorities, too. They follow a specific protocol during a crisis. In an emergency (perceived or real), the body goes into high gear: It invokes the fight-or-flight response. All resources (brain function, blood flow, strength/muscle capacity) go into survival mode.

A man chased by a wild animal exhibits fight-or-flight characteristics. He doesn't take time to pull a few weeds along the way. His physical and mental capabilities work at their peak, in tandem, to overcome the crisis.

For some of us with chronic illnesses, the fight-or-flight mode becomes continuously engaged. Whether from prolonged illness, family crisis, or post-traumatic stress syndrome, the body is stuck in fight-or-flight status. One casualty of this scenario you might not consider is digestion.

Your body's job of digesting food is as fundamental as breathing. When you're under emotional duress — whether waiting for the sky to fall or the forty days of rain to stop — your body is busy doing other things. There's no time to digest the mondo burger, curly fries, and shake that you consumed. Instead, your lunch sits in an acidic stomach (increased acid is another side effect of fight-or-flight), waiting for available resources.

When the body gets stuck in this pattern, it plays the same tune over and over, like the skipping needle on a vinyl record. The long-term effects are devastating.

Your state of mind plays a crucial role in your healthy future. What fears, anxieties, or stresses govern your emotional state? Are you too busy running from danger to make an assessment?

When you unravel the emotional stressors that keep you stuck in the fight-or-flight mode, you'll free up your body's resources for other activities, including healthier digestion. This is one instance where unraveling is a *good* thing.

FOR WHOM THE WELL TOLLS

Staying well isn't easy, especially when chronic illness gets in the way. Oftentimes, the difference between well and unwell is one small word: *no*.

The average parent's life is full of choices. School activities and community events compete with work and household responsibilities.

Lines blur. How often do you say *yes* when you want to say *no* when asked to volunteer? For some, saying *no* is easy; for others, it takes a toll. For people-pleasers (like me), saying *no* leaves a well of guilt and frustration. We say *yes* because we know we can do what's asked of us. Our *yes* response isn't based on availability or even desire, but instead purely on our competency.

Obligations are double-edged. Added commitments become a heavy burden. Saying *no* leads to conflicting emotions: That's burdensome, too.

No is not a bad thing. Don't think of your next refusal as a failure. Think of it as self-preservation. If *you* don't take steps to protect your health, *who will*?

I struggled with the adult onset of "should" for many years. I *should* volunteer as room mom and participate in every vocal and instrumental opportunity available. In my former "should days," I worked full-time, attended school part-time, cared for a house, spouse, and kids, all while juggling rehearsals and board meetings.

> "*A* strong positive mental attitude will create more miracles than any wonder drug."
>
> —Patricia Neal

Predictably, the activities took a toll. For me, the evening activities were the worst. I paid a physical price the following day (or days). Still, I didn't listen to my own body.

I didn't react until my choices disappeared. When chronic illness knocked me flat, my shoulds turned into can'ts.

If this has happened to you, take a look at which activities sap your energy and which replenish it. We can't avoid every energy-sapping activity, but becoming selective is a great place to start.

WHAT'S YOUR I.T.M.?

Stress is palpable as it sinks into our muscles, bones, and gut. That feeling is tension. For most of my adult life, my inner tension level was as taut as a piano wire. That was my "normal." The first time I did a round of MTT (Meridian Tapping Technique), I remember feeling calm, tingly, and slightly empty, as if something was absent from the pit of my stomach. Later, I recognized that I felt the same way after tai chi.

I eventually recognized the feeling as the *absence* of tension. Stress and its byproduct, tension, were so familiar that I only noticed their absence, not their presence.

It took practice to identify the levels of my inner tension. I had to remind myself (frequently!) to take a deep breath and kick my inner idle into low gear. I call it my *inner tension meter* (I.T.M.). When stressed, I feel my tension ratchet up. When I feel it increasing, I take action: deep breaths, a change of scenery, a hot bath, exercise, or a cup of tea. If the situation warrants, I also employ prayer, MTT, or other relaxation methods. Sometimes it takes a combination of healing modalities.

Inner tension may sound minor, but, over time, stress corrodes your digestive health and impairs your immune system, leaving you vulnerable to secondary illnesses.

The next time you feel your I.T.M. spike, take action. Apply relaxation methods liberally until symptoms abate. That's a wellness prescription with no co-pay required.

PICK A BUDDY BOUQUET

Good friends are the floating rafts in the swimming pool of life. They're the daisies in our daisy-chain necklace. There's nothing like laughing at a shared, inside joke with someone who truly "gets" you. In the interest of rebuilding wellness, it's important to surround yourself with others who share similar ideals and goals.

It's a two-way street. When others bless us, they receive supportive energy in return. We're lucky if we have one true friend who fits this category.

Not everyone is as helpful as a true friend. We have to find healthy ways to deal with acquaintances, friends, family, and coworkers who fall short (either a little or a lot) of being helpful.

One way to evaluate a true friend is to inventory your energy state after a visit. Do you feel invigorated? Mellow? Sucked dry as a bathtub after the plug is pulled?

I've finally given myself permission to admit that some people are simply annoying (including some I care about). Their negative mood no longer impacts mine as it used to. I take a deep breath and smile, knowing their issues are not my issues, and vice versa.

I don't necessarily avoid negative people, but I've taken myself off the hook for trying to please them. We have to work with all types of people, and it's a disservice to let their negativity leave a physical impact.

Taking a step back helps in another way, too. When you're no longer trying to solve someone else's problems, you're in a better position to listen. Maybe that's what was needed in the first place.

In the end, only people of our choosing have influence over us, and, even then, only if we let them. True friends, of course, are forever arranged in our buddy bouquets.

MEMENTO MEMORIES

It doesn't take much to spur a pleasant memory. A favorite frosting-scented lotion reminds me of my sisters. I carry a purse from a thoughtful daughter. Because I'm a reader, I've repurposed keepsakes as bookmarks, including a tag from a doll store, a centennial banquet place card, and many airline, movie, and symphony tickets. For me, it's fitting for items that carry fond memories to hold a place in my books — where I see them most.

Mementos can evoke a sense of peace. In Honolulu, I found a paperback-width cardstock note slipped under my hotel room door. Waves of aqua blue fade into a cream sea speckled with random Japanese text. Loosely translated it says: "I've been to your room, but I respected your privacy. I am therefore disappointed in my inability to clean it. Sincerely, Your Housekeeper."

It makes a great bookmark and simply glancing at that card

gives me a sense of serenity. I finger the worn edges and recall that somewhere in the world exists *My Housekeeper*. She's bereft in her disappointment.

Each time I see it, I'm reminded that my care was once someone else's top priority. That's enough to make me sigh.

Do you have mementos that make you sigh, smile, or fill you with sense of peace? Carry them with you as a talisman or remembrance of well-being. Feeling good is not a state of mind, but your state of mind *can* help you feel good.

"A man too busy to care for his health is like a craftsman too busy to care for his tools."

—Spanish Proverb

Chapter 8

How I Lost My Balance but Gained a Spine

think of this chapter as I do my kitchen junk drawer — important stuff that's hard to categorize. My junk drawer contains otherwise homeless utensils, gadgets, and doohickeys. The sections in this chapter may seem random, but they demonstrate how the individual components of the restoration trio work together.

Like my junk drawer, this is the go-to place for all things miscellaneous.

SPIRALING INTO CONTROL

Components of the restoration trio are equally important, but I've presented them in the same order and emphasis as my experiences.

It took me longer to accept "we are what we eat" than to accept the truths about exercise and emotional wellness. I'm not alone. Food is a touchy subject. I've found that suggesting alternative food choices to a hungry woman is like poking a cub in front of mama bear. Not always wise.

If you're a "mama bear" and find yourself defending, arguing, or struggling with suggested nutritional ideas, that's okay. Take time to review Chapter Five and do research on your own. Let ideas sink in. Go at your own pace. Above all, be kind to yourself (I can't say that enough).

The concept of exercise doesn't seem to suffer the same stigma. Society generally accepts that exercise is a good idea. You might drag your feet with the execution of the advice, but the advice itself isn't threatening. The same goes for emotional wellness and stress-relieving activities. Who doesn't agree that reduced stress is desirable? It stands to reason, therefore, that dietary changes may take longer to implement.

Seeking wellness is a unifying goal. Identifying your personal "weakest link" helps you set priorities. If the thought of changing your eating habits makes you dig in your heels in protest, begin there. If exercise seems too big, too difficult, or impossible, take small steps. If you're overworked and overstressed, say hello to yoga and tai chi for starters. Whatever your needs, set wellness as a priority and move forward.

I've always thought of the healing path as a spiral. It's a common symbol found in nature. I loved the concept of spirals so much that *Spiraling INTO Control* was the working title of this book for many years. Unique as snowflakes and fingerprints, spirals represent the individual journey. Everyone's spiral path is different. Forward motion is the only requirement. Even *one step* from where you are is progress.

Life experiences provide learning opportunities along the way. We learn, trip, fall, get up, and learn again. That's the journey. Spirals show us that we're not the center of the universe. Each person begins from a different place. The goal is to focus on our own journey rather than on another's.

The spiral journey works like a centrifuge, putting a spin and emphasis on what's important. Looking within helps to sort things without. That's the spiral of life.

Oh, and about control? It's what we all seek and crave. The concept of control is attractive, but healing is not, and has never been, about control. Acceptance is a far better concept.

Your healing path begins with you. Where do you place your needs on your spiral path? If you say you'll get well someday, that's exactly when it will happen.

And, someday is never today.

ço

I'm not the same person I was at the beginning of my health journey. A decade ago, I was physically and mentally dizzy. I didn't know truth from fiction. Today, I'm neither passive nor helpless. I'm more centered and aware of what I want. I'm equally aware of what I don't want. Those who truly care for me embrace the changes. Others aren't so happy with the "new" me. They've found fault in my decisions, chastised me for my choices. They're offended that my response to their *jump* request is no longer *how high*.

Life-altering change begins with a thought. A niggling idea that seems contrary to what you believe about yourself. For me, it was the notion I could actively rebuild wellness. Who was I to choose a different path from the one paved by the traditional medical community? Could I really question established protocol?

Self-education is the key to success. Learn about your health issues. Take charge! Don't expect anyone else to care as much as you. Learn to read your body's clues. What feels nourishing? What feels soul-sucking? If a health professional tells you something that doesn't sound right to you, ask questions. If that upsets him or her, move on. Your health is at stake, and you deserve answers.

Before I paint an embellished portrait of myself as always confident and focused, I must confess. I'm still a hopeless rule-follower. I constantly seek the approval of others, my true nature. But I have learned this: I color outside the lines when necessary.

I've realized that wellness requires activity and action. Passively seeking wellness fails to bring results. I lost my balance many times on my journey toward wellness, but falling wasn't as hard as deciding to get back up.

VOTER EDUCATION

Elections pop up around my area more often than bank holidays. *Vote for Me* signs sprout across lawns; pamphlets multiply in mailboxes, and TV pitches blur the airwaves. I stack snail mail voting information in one place (like a tote bag) and sort through it before voting day. I read the materials (paying attention to the "paid by" committee), go online for additional information, and make calls if necessary.

By the time I cast my vote I've done my research and feel I can make an intelligent decision. Tossing all the campaign propaganda is my favorite part of voting day! But what if I had to vote again the following week? Would I remember who I voted for? Probably. But would I remember the details of the obscure local propositions? Probably not.

I approach many medical decisions in the same way. I do my research, make my decision, and move on. I'm often asked for my opinion on what types of supplements I use or what treatments work for me. I can explain why I follow one protocol or another, but

I can't always recall the details that helped me reach my conclusion.

My brain is over-capacity when it comes to knowing the milligrams of magnesium I consume, or the details of how hormones regulate the metabolism. I could claim this tendency to be a symptom of fibro fog, but anyone's brain can suffer system overload from such minutia.

The old adage, "The devil is in the details," applies here. Details assist in helping make the decision, but once it's made? Let go!

MY WINDOW OF WELL

Fibromyalgia distills the truth with an undeniable clarity. When first diagnosed, I realized my body's "needs" overruled my mind's "wants." It wasn't a fair fight. At first I denied my physical limitations and resented my uncooperative body. I tried to do everything as I had before. Working against my limitations simply increased my symptoms: more pain, fatigue, dizziness. I wasn't listening to what my body had to say.

Slowly, I began to weed out activities. I dropped choirs, instrumental groups, board positions, and social commitments. I sent myself mental *I'm sorry for your loss* cards and attended my own protracted pity party.

In time, my increased energy surprised me. I noticed that when I didn't zap my resources (with evening activities), I experienced improved sleep. I awoke feeling refreshed and considered it an accomplishment. I felt less sloth, more jackrabbit.

I term my hours of peak operation my "window of well." Though I get up early most mornings, it may take hours for the stiffness to go away. This is my burnoff point (as discussed in Chapter Three). I feel my best from about ten a.m. to four p.m. When my window of well closes, stiffness creeps back in, and fatigue makes a house call.

This is only *my* window of well; everyone's window will vary. I have friends with chronic fatigue, rheumatoid arthritis, lupus, or cancer who've adopted their own window of well principle. They respect their physical rhythms and work within them, when possible. Some sleep 'til noon and then feel "ablaze" 'til midnight. Because sleep disorders are so prevalent with chronic illness, it's not unusual to find fibrofolk asleep at one in the afternoon and vacuuming the house at one in the morning. They're operating within their current window of well.

Fibromyalgia has turned me into a desert bloom. I open midmorning and close tight before sundown. I've learned to respect my window of well and, rather than resenting the activities I'm missing, perspective allows me to give thanks for the bloomin' time I have!

NUTRITIONAL RESUMÉ

Think about your favorite room. What makes it your favorite? Wall color, textures, art, decorator items? It may not be magazine perfect, but it's the true you.

Now think about yesterday. What did you put inside your body from dawn to dusk? What does that reflect? Did you select foods that reflect the true you?

These were my thoughts as I sat one rainy afternoon at Starbucks waiting for my writer's group. I saw a woman exit her gleaming SUV (sport utility vehicle). Her appearance was so ostentatious, she seemed to glide in slow motion.

First, one magnificent stiletto-heeled boot dipped beneath the door. A large tortoiseshell buckle graced the ankle with champagne-colored suede extending up to the knee. Footwear better suited for catwalks than sidewalks. Emerging farther, I saw a short, fashionable trench coat belted snugly over an equally fashionable outfit.

She was dressed for success. Her trendy attire painted a picture of financial affluence. But her order, a frothy latte with caramel syrup and whipped cream and an oversized muffin, prompted me to wonder: Did she care as much for the inside of her body as for the outside?

My husband watches stock market channels twenty-four-seven. The phrase "a healthy bottom line" is often linked to financial security. Frequent deposits and careful monitoring of accounts assures financial success.

But what about nutritional security? Why aren't we as careful with the deposits we make to our health accounts?

Eating well today is akin to financially investing in your future. It's equally, if not more, important an investment than funding your 401(k) or IRA. Who wants riches in assets but poverty in health? We all know people who've scrimped and saved for retirement only to spend their hard-earned savings on unplanned medical costs.

Based on Ms. Trenchcoat's appearance, I believe her business resumè is probably impressive. Based on her behaviors, it's less likely that her nutritional resumè is impressive. Yes, she can be healthy and have her calorie-laden latte. She might be a yoga instructor who "eats clean" ninety percent of the time. But, it's also possible that her nutritional "savings" are in danger of dipping into the red.

Think about the deposits you make to your nutritional accounts. Healthy deposits today compound exponentially toward a healthy future — a tip you can take to the bank. Your insides deserve as much care as your outsides. Investing in good food today pays dividends far into your healthy future.

KIKI DEE PERSPECTIVE

Radio dedications used to be a commonplace teenage experience, but not in the itty-bitty hamlet of my youth. Located half a state away, only one rock and roll station existed in the whole of Iowa.

In my junior year of high school, I learned a neighboring school was hosting a dance and live radio broadcast. Promised a song dedication from friends, I waited at home to hear my boyfriend's name entwined with mine. When it happened, the accompanying song surprised me. I expected *When I Need You* by Leo Sayer or *Muskrat Love* by the Captain & Tennille. Instead, Elton John and Kiki Dee's *Don't Go Breakin' My Heart* played to the rhythm of my own wildly thumping heart.

Hmm … why did my friends choose *that* song to represent my forever love match? I never asked. I probably didn't want to know.

The truth is that my friends had perspective. They saw my darling boyfriend for what he was — a player. Unfortunately, I had to realize that much later for myself. I needed distance and time to gain perspective.

Because friends know you best, enlist them as part of your better health team. Tell them your plans. Friends can spot the chinks in your armor. They may be your best source for ideas on how to achieve your goals. Objectivity gives them perspective.

Perspective combined with distance can be enlightening. I once saw my own home from my neighbor's dining room window. My house looked strange, almost foreign. I noticed the stucco wall needed paint and what an eyesore the stuff "stored" near the garage had become. This neighborly perspective gave a different view.

Listen to your friends' perspective. They can give you a different view of something you may be too close to see. If you're concerned they'll sabotage your progress, then I suggest you get new friends. True friends share in successes. In any case, you get to choose how to react to their comments.

I can only suggest you listen to their perspective and give it a little more thought than, hmm....

ROSE BUDS VS. TASTE BUDS

We all like to feel appreciated. When you want to shower someone with gratitude, what gifts or gestures come to mind?

For most of us, the first response is something edible. Candy, baked goods, or chocolate shows appreciation, right? Friends, teachers, coworkers, ministers, neighbors, healthcare workers — they all *deserve* something good.

We need to alter our belief systems, to change our expectation of "good." We need to change how we show appreciation. Teachers have confessed to me immense guilt over throwing away tins of homemade cookies and boxes of chocolates. Is that how we want to make them feel?

This topic came up recently, at a party-planning meeting for a deserving volunteer. A large sheet cake and other sugary goodies were discussed. I stated desserts might not be the best way to show appreciation. (Everyone in the group, including the honoree, suffers from chronic illnesses.) I made several alternative suggestions that were quickly overruled.

Frustrated, I helped pass out slabs of cake at that event. I heard a flurry of comments such as, "Oh, I shouldn't," "My ankles are gonna swell tomorrow from this but, oh well," and, "I'll have just a bite, since they went to all this trouble."

It felt like I was handing out shots of whiskey at an A.A. meeting.

Knowing the intention was good, I said nothing more. We honored a lovely lady.

I would have preferred to honor her with handwritten notes, flowers, gift cards, or perhaps a certificate for a massage or spa date. Appreciation can take place in other tangible, healthy ways. Truth is, gifts don't need to contain sugar to garner the response, "How sweet!"

EAT NOW!

I used to think that Norwegians were famous for eating. Every holiday and get-together focused on two things: what's for supper, and when is supper? "Eat now!" was our call to arms (of the cutlery variety).

I now understand that food worship knows no border. Every ethnicity has its own culinary delights and devotions; comfort foods exist everywhere. At my childhood home, Thanksgiving dinners weren't complete without buttered kringla and sugared lefse. Other cultures may have empanadas, baklava, hummus and pitas, roast duck with shiitake mushroom gravy, or tandoori chicken and chutney.

I used to think of comfort foods as indulgences. They were foods not necessarily good for me but those that make me feel good. Sadly, the "good" feeling was fleeting, and the lasting effects were not.

I grew up. Comfort foods mean something different now. I seek foods that comfort by nourishing and sustaining me — without regret. I've broadened my dietary horizons to include foods from all over the world, picking the best choices for my family and me. Now *that's* comforting.

I encourage you to take a second look at what foods give you comfort. It's a fabulous, multi-cultural culinary world out there. What stews in your kitchen's melting pot?

MONTE CRISTO IS MORE THAN A SANDWICH

There are few movies that I'll watch repeatedly. The 2002 film *The Count of Monte Cristo* is a family favorite. The complex storyline of the classic novel highlights the virtue of patience and planning. In a favorite scene, a jumpy sidekick listens to the count's intricate plot for revenge and blurts, "Why not just kill them? I'll run up to Paris — bam, bam, bam, bam. I'm back before week's end. We spend the treasure. How is this a bad plan?"

He failed to grasp the importance of patience.

The Count of Monte Cristo was all about patience and planning. He had nothing but time when imprisoned in Chateau d'If (France's Alcatraz). Upon his escape, he envisioned the benefits of a well-thought-out plan.

Whenever my husband or I want to forgo planning for expediency, the other teases, "Bam, bam. How is this a bad plan?"

"Plan" is my favorite four-letter word. Happenstance and serendipity are my acquaintances, but *plan* is my new BFF. Lifestyle changes take planning. No plan = no action. No action = no opportunity for success.

Eating well takes planning, on the road and at home. When did you last read the menu at Wanna Burger Now? Are there healthier alternatives? Go menu spelunking. Talk to your server about substitutions and menu options. I learned from a helpful server that I can order "double salad, no rice" at my favorite Greek restaurant. Talk about win/win. I skip the over processed rice and get twice as much salad for the same price.

I've learned to scour the ingredients and nutrition listings (if available) of my favorite menu items. They're not always as healthy as they appear. I discovered that a health watchdog site voted my all-time favorite salad, "Saltiest in America." Yikes! Digging a little further online, the abundance of data available surprised me. Nutritional statistics exist on many restaurant chain websites or from sites such as http://www.calorieking. com/ and http://www.nutritiondata. com/. In fact, if nutritional data is unavailable for a restaurant, I'd suggest a boycott. What are they hiding?

> "*Life is a continuous exercise in creative problem-solving.*"
> —Michael J. Gelb

Again, planning comes to the rescue. I can order that super-salty salad sans the saltiest ingredients and portion it by asking for a take-home box right away. Another good idea is to order items without the tempting sides. Order "no fries, please" rather than falling prey to "It *comes* with fries anyway. I'll just have a couple."

I'm also fond of B.Y.O.V. (bring your own veggies). It's the doggy-bag scenario in reverse. I bring small baggies of spinach, chopped broccoli, or diced peppers to add to my entree. Some healthy foods can be quite portable. I love veggies: no drug interaction concerns, no freakish side effects.

Planning nutritious meals at home is even easier. After produce shopping, chop the veggies right away. Putting them into small bags or containers keeps them handy for soups, salads, wraps, omelets, chili, crockpot meals, or pitas. I add chopped veggies to meatloaf and burger patties as well as sauces and eggs. Having chopped veggies at the ready makes it easy to amp up daily servings.

Planning healthy meals starts at the grocery store. Fill your cart with fresh produce and foods such as beans, eggs, organic broths, and quality meats (if you desire). From my experience, eating healthy is a money saver. Yes, you read that correctly. I rarely buy frozen or expensive pre-packaged foods. I also have no use for Big Bulk Stores. Amazing but true. I found that when I don't push that gigantic cart around the gigantic store, I don't have gigantic food bills.

After all, how many items on my last Big Bulk Store receipt were truly food-related? Did I really need that mondo blow-up floating recliner for the pool? Wait a minute ... I don't even have a pool!

If only I'd planned for the future like the Count of Monte Cristo....

MY HUNGRY GIRL

We've rescued two Shelties (Shetland sheepdogs). Our first beautiful girl, Shelby, had issues. Her hunger knew no bounds. Hunger existed in every hair, whisker, and toenail of her being. Her actions spoke loudly; she behaved as though she were starving to death.

She came to us at forty-six pounds with strict orders from the vet to reduce that by half. The night we brought her home, she ate her dinner and the takeout trash from ours. When she threw up later (we learned this was part of her routine), the sandwich shop logo still glistened legibly on the napkins. She rarely chewed.

Shelby found her nutritious meals wholly unsatisfying. Within weeks, she scavenged six-dozen peanut-butter cookies (including paper plates and bags), a five-pound bag of flour, candles, lotions, toothpaste, soap, cough drops, candies, lip balm, chocolates, and minted dental floss.

If it had a scent, she ate it.

This grossly overweight dog couldn't jump onto the sofa, yet telltale paw prints graced the *top* of the dining room table. She licked the butter dish clean, later leaving a greasy calling card on my new bedspread. She was a canine bulimic.

Her soft brown eyes said, "I can't help it," but something deeper brewed. She wasn't hungry; she was angry-hungry. She gobbled every morsel as if fearing a permanently empty bowl. We prohibited hand-feeding for anyone wishing to keep all digits intact.

I learned that Shelby suffered from severe abandonment issues. Foods could not heal her emotional wounds. Using foods as a placeholder for an emotional lack is familiar for people, too.

Hunger pangs may prompt you to ask, "What do I *really* want?"

Luck is on your side. You're not a canine and can figure out the origins of your hunger issues. Ask yourself a few questions before you grab a snack. Am I truly hungry, or am I trying to fill an emotional void? Is this nourishing?

Your answers may be surprising. Some people are unaware of their inner chatter. Subliminal thoughts about not being good enough or thin enough are common. MTT can prove very helpful at dealing with negative self-talk.

One of the phrases or affirmations I try to focus on is the word *enough*. This meal is enough. My actions are enough. I am enough. After all, the opposite of enough — lack or deprivation — drives people to do unhealthy things. In this abundant society, we are neither lacking nor deprived, yet that inner feeling lingers. We think, if three cookies are good, the entire package is better.

Digging into the garden of your psyche may help you unearth the source of your hunger. Once you've revealed it, looked at it, and dealt with it, you'll gain a peaceful resonance with the word "enough." You'll find that *enough* satisfies every hunger.

A ROSE BY ANY OTHER NAME CAN STILL STINK

Lots of things stink: foods, cleaning products, home-improvement products, plastic wrappers, deodorizers, perfumes, and scented candles. Just as beauty is in the eye of the beholder, stink is in the nose of the sniffer. A pleasant odor for one might be a harmful assault for another.

Cigarette smoke is lethal-smelling to me. I can discern if a first-time acquaintance is a smoker or if he simply carpooled with one. Either way, a prompt headache is my reward for sharing his air space.

Sensory ultra-sensitivity is a fibromyalgia theme. All the senses are subject to over-stimulation: touch, sound, smell, light, taste. Some fibrofolk can't tolerate bright lights or loud sounds. Chemical-laden foods and smells are problematic for many.

Finding out what's toxic can be confusing. It'd be nice if hazardous products were clearly labeled. A neon orange "Beware of Poison" sticker complete with a skull and crossbones on room deodorizers would suffice. Seemingly innocuous household products can be harmful — to us as well as to the environment. Think of the perfumed items in your home. Soaps, lotions, tissues, detergents, deodorizers, and candles all use masking scents. Without the added "fresh" smell, all that's left is the enticing aroma of a chemistry lab.

Reading the labels on household supplies is as important as for food. If possible, give a product the sniff test before you buy. Listen to your body. Take note of your reaction(s). Does one whiff seem to hit you between the eyes? Does the odor tie your stomach in a knot?

I once became ill from driving a rental car. The rental agent proudly plopped the keys in my palm stating, "You don't know the hoops I jumped through for you. It's only got twelve miles on it." I didn't have the heart to tell him I don't like "new-car smell." Inside the car, my head felt swimmy and thick. I drove the "toxic taxi" for three days before I cried uncle. Foggy and overwhelmed, I became lost in a familiar neighborhood. After finding the rental agency, I sprinted from the car as if it were in flames. I tossed the keys on the counter and said, "Give me something old and well-ventilated."

Due to these ultra-sensitivities, fibrofolk are today's coal mine canaries.

I wish we could put our "gift" to good use without negatively impacting our health. If so, we could earn a living as paid "bio hazard specialists." We could visit areas of suspected toxic contamination while scientists documented our progress:

- Marked decrease in cognitive skills performance.
- Hand-eye coordination failure.
- Central nervous system impact likely.
- Conclusion: toxic contamination probable.

I'm using hyperbole here, but, unfortunately, some fibrofolk live out this scenario in reality. Working or living in toxic buildings or near substances such as paints, dyes, and pesticides can result in immune system overload. For a short time, I worked for a silk-screening company and breathed my share of noxious ink fumes. I had little awareness then of the effects of my personal surroundings. I understood neither the impact of the toxins, nor the extent of my already compromised health. I only knew that my illness progressed rapidly during the time I worked there.

Whether respect for your air space is familiar territory or a newly developed skill, take the time to surround yourself with a sweet-smelling, natural, healthful environment.

Stop and smell the roses.

DOES THIS HAND LOTION COME IN OTHER FLAVORS?

Imagine this: Step into your shower, remove the cap from your favorite hair conditioner and take a swig.

Other than in extreme cases of sleepwalking disorders, it's not likely anyone would purposely ingest hair care products. You may not think you "consume" beauty products, but you do. Your skin is your body's largest organ. Your skin holds the good stuff in and helps to keep the bad stuff out. Like M&M's® candy coating, skin is your body's first line of protection.

Skin needs all the assistance it can get. Consider carefully what you put *on* your body. Skin care products, makeup, lotions, and deodorants don't simply float on the surface. What you put onto your skin seeps into tissues and the bloodstream. Do your skin care products contain healthy and natural ingredients? Do they come from trustworthy sources?

Avoid potentially harmful ingredients such as parabens, petroleum, propylene glycol, aluminum, mineral oil, synthetic fillers, urea, phthalates, artificial dyes, fragrances, and talc.

It's easier than ever to comparison shop. The natural skin care market has exploded over the past decade, increasing awareness. Look for products that contain safe, non-toxic, organic, and botanically-based ingredients for you and your family. Read the label on the product itself *and* don't forget the fine print inside the packaging. Sometimes, the most important information is in the smallest type.

Use sunscreen cautiously. It's no coincidence that the rate of skin cancer has *increased* with the rate of sunscreen use. Hand sanitizers, too, often contain harmful ingredients. Although it may take a bit of sleuthing, natural alternatives are available.

If a hair care or skin care product isn't something you'd put in your mouth, reconsider putting it on your skin.

MED-ITATIONS

I searched for pain relief for many years. I indiscriminately consumed as directed any prescribed medications. I took muscle relaxers, anti-inflammatories, anti-depressants (part of IBS protocol), serotonin-leveling meds, and Cox-2 inhibitors. I did find some pain relief and thought the meds gave me the edge to manage my symptoms.

> "*When solving problems, dig at the roots instead of just hacking at the leaves.*"
>
> —Anthony J. D'Angelo

I won't deny another fact. Taking prescribed medications made me feel validated. It felt as if someone "out there" listened and took my pain seriously. I had a doctor-certified diagnosis, and his white square of paper offered a solution. That prescription was my square stamp of hope — proof that something was wrong.

As I began to understand myself better, my need to feel validated by others lessened. I no longer needed anyone else's "seal of approval." It mattered little what anyone else thought.

As my nutrition and exercise regimen became integral to

my life, my dependence on meds decreased. The "as needed" medications simply weren't needed at all. Others — some I'd been on for years — I weaned off slowly, <u>with my doctor's observation and approval</u>. I tracked my progress on a calendar, expecting to feel my pain increase as my medications decreased. That didn't happen. In fact, as I continued with my holistic regimen, my pain levels continued to decrease. Headaches and the burning/tingling pain in my fingertips disappeared almost completely.

To clarify: This was MY path. I don't suggest altering medication regimens for anyone else. *Never* discontinue medications without first discussing it with your doctor. I can only convey my experiences. I'm certain that healthy eating and regular exercise played a primary role in the rehabilitation of my digestive system and my body.

From time to time, I experience symptom flare-ups, mostly attributed to outside factors such as family, work, and changes in what I eat. I can predict with fair accuracy when I've done something that will cause increased pain or fatigue. Now, I'm in a good position to mitigate those flare-ups: They have no power over me.

All I can say is that it's great to be in the driver's seat!

MONEY THROUGH FRIDAY

Goin' green doesn't mean goin' broke. Don't believe me? Healthy foods are often inexpensive. Consider this: Where do you find bags of dried lentils, pintos, kidney, and navy beans at the grocery store? They reside on the bottom shelves along with other lower-priced goods. Products with the fattest profit margins are stocked at eye level. By simply shopping "below the belt," you can make your grocery budget go further.

Beans top the bargain list due to their "big bang for the buck" quality. Providing protein, fiber, and other essential nutrients, beans stretch a dollar a long way. One bag can make a large pot of soup or chili that can extend to multiple servings.

Another great bargain comes from the produce section. Vegetables are typically inexpensive, depending on the variety and the store. I've come home from local farmer's markets with several bags of produce for under ten dollars. Shop within season, when possible, for the freshest and healthiest choices. In metropolitan areas, fruits and vegetables are available year 'round, but take into consideration the environmental impact of imported produce. I'm less likely to make a purchase if I believe the fruit or vegetable came by boat from another country.

I have a friend who calls her thrifty shopping techniques "perimeter shopping." She only makes purchases from the produce section and from select areas along the outside walls of the store. The interior sections of most markets contain the processed foods. All that packaging, production, and top-dollar marketing adds up to pricey products. The basic ingredients may be cheap, but by the time they're combined into a slick and hyped-up product, the price soars.

I recently participated in a food drive for a local food bank. A pre-printed list was provided, and filling my cart with the requested items frustrated me. Not only were the choices unhealthy, they were unnecessarily expensive. I could have purchased more (not to mention healthier) food for fewer dollars.

Foods with less packaging cost less and create less waste. Less waste means less trash to the curb and less trash taken to landfills.

The stigma that all healthy foods are expensive comes, in part, from those opposed to the organic industry. Organic products are often pricier than those not certified. They are non-GMO foods (GMO – genetically modified organisms). Organic produce is grown without chemicals such as pesticides or herbicides. Organic livestock is reared without the use of antibiotics or growth hormones.

Some produce should be bought as organic and is worth the premium price. Non-organic pears, apples, strawberries, spinach, peppers, and imported grapes may contain high levels of pesticides. Of course, local farmer's markets are always the best solutions for fresh produce unless you plant your own garden. It's generally thought that meat and dairy products are almost always worth the upgraded price to buy organic. Knowing the origins of your food is worth the effort.

By the way, it's okay to throw away produce you didn't "get to" before it went bad. It was still a good investment. I'd rather toss a pound of produce than keep ten pounds of processed junk. You're still dollars (and "wellth") ahead.

Eating healthier means saving money. This has been my experience even considering the higher prices of organic foods. My overall grocery bills have decreased significantly in recent years due to changed eating habits. This saving extends even further when adding reduced healthcare costs to the equation. A healthier immune system means fewer co-pays and doctor office visits.

So what do I do, you may wonder, with all the money I save by eating healthy and staying well? That's funny. My husband wants to know the same thing.

SEW YOUR WILD OATS – OR BARLEY

I always say that my personal thermostat is broken. My body temperature vacillates between toasty and freezing with not much middle ground. Whether thyroid or hormone-related, I lack the ability to consistently regulate my internal temperature. Needing clothes suitable for both Honolulu and Anchorage poses a problem. I simplify by wearing them all at once. I've been known to wear shorts, a tank top, socks, and a wool scarf.

Chronic illness couture is unique. Comfort trumps fashion every time. Leather coats give way to bathrobes, pumps to slippers. For extra warmth, lots of fibrofolk use heating pads, but I find the electrical cord a nuisance. Instead, I tend to wear vests and clothes in layers. I may look as if I share a tailor with Tevye from *Fiddler on the Roof*, but it works for me.

I love scarves. Wearing one is both a fashion statement and a band-aid for what ails me. I consider them portable, temporary turtlenecks. Just a little bit of warmth where I need it — and simple to remove when I don't. From thick wool to lightweight eyelash yarn, they're superior to too-heavy gel-filled pads.

I've tried about every organic hot/cold pack I can find. Most are filled with dense contents: flax, rice, corn, beans, etc. My shoulders ache more from the hot pack than from fibromyalgia. Years ago, at a local craft fair, I found a not-so-heavy, simple tube-type neck wrap. Filled with barley, it's both inexpensive and lightweight. Sold.

As a fibromyalgia fashion plate, I wear scarves, vests, hot packs, and wooly blankets. I often wear sweaters with one sleeve on. On chilly evenings, I'm likely wearing one fuzzy sock.

What works for you? Whatever you wear, do it with confidence and don't worry. Obscurity has its benefits. Mr. Blackwell isn't likely to care.

SLEEP PERCHANCE TO CATCH SOME MUCH NEEDED Z'S

In Chapter Three, I said that when your life is balanced (nutrition, exercise, emotional wellness), sleep follows. Here's why:

People dealing with fibromyalgia, chronic fatigue, and other related disorders are understandably *desperate* for sleep solutions. My sleepless nights went on for more than fifteen years. The more I chased sleep, the further out of reach it dangled.

I put the cart before the horse—looking for sleep when my body looked for wholeness.

Sleep became almost the last health puzzle piece to fall into place. But once fixed, it stayed fixed. Now, sleepless nights seldom occur and clearly relate to stress and/or not enough exercise.

When the body's basic needs are met through proper nutrition, daily movement, and emotional wellness, sleep is a natural byproduct. Sleep (and proper sleep hygiene) helps to repair, rejuvenate, and renew the body. It'll happen when you actively take steps to repair what is broken. My sister says that fixing chronic illness is like trying to turn around the *Titanic*. Yes, it's tough, but it gets easier as we learn to detect and dodge the icebergs.

> "*Sleep is the golden chain that ties health and our bodies together.*"
>
> —Thomas Dekker

I repaired nutritional damage to my body and then added exercise and stress-relieving modalities. Repairing my body nutritionally (including replenishing vitamins and minerals) became the foundation of what I needed. I was ready for the next step. After a healthy workout, I had my *first* taste of a good night's sleep. There was a direct connection. Because regular exercise is linked to catching those Z's, I spell sleep, S-W-E-A-T!

FOURTEEN CARROT GOALS

I'm a fan of setting goals. Whether major (i.e., writing five-hundred words per day) or minor (folding laundry), goal-setting is good mental exercise.

Recently, I jotted down a to-do list for one Friday. I had fourteen separate tasks, some quickies, some not. I realized as I estimated times for each, that my list was unrealistic. I had to re-think and re-prioritize. If I hadn't put it in writing, I would have rushed around all day with my mental to-do list, feeling frazzled and unproductive.

Before you let your plans go all hinky, take another look. Are you trying to squeeze too much into your window of well? Are your daily goals realistic?

Memory issues aside, putting pen to paper helps to categorize tasks. It's an easy way to prioritize. Listing goals has another benefit. Once completed, checking them off is bliss!

Think of the list as a goal-setting nudge, something to get you started. Don't forget to set rewards for a job well done. If you have difficulty in coming up with your goals list, try the following:

- Be specific. Break down your goals into finite tasks.
  (*Sort junk mail/load dishwasher* rather than *clean kitchen*.)
- Make lists and sub-lists if necessary.
  (*Finish Office Project: 1- Research, 2- Organize research notes, 3- Write report*.)
- Write a free-form goals list, including all goals, thoughts, ideas. From this list, use a highlighter to pinpoint commonalities and themes. Consolidate these ideas into your main goals list, or use it as is.
- List rewards as well as goals.
  (Include rewards unrelated to food.)

Using the goal-and-reward method of accomplishing tasks takes thought at first, but becomes second nature. A goals list is not static; it's ever-changing. Keep pen and paper handy to jot down goals and rewards as they pop up.

You'll know you're in control when you become adept at motivating yourself. Dangle your own carrots!

PLEASE EXCUSE CATHY....

A few months after I spoke on the topic of nutrition at a fibromyalgia support group, Cathy asked me to lunch. We'd barely arrived when she began peppering me with nutrition questions. It was clear she'd been doing research and trying new things based on my advice.

She poured out a litany of failed attempts at reshaping her eating habits. She confessed gargantuan efforts and abysmal defeats. I suggested alternatives for each circumstance.

Noticeably annoyed, she said, "You have an answer for everything; don't you!"

Isn't that what she asked for?

Poking angrily at her salad, she changed the subject to generalities; kids, house, and pets.

It dawned on me later that she didn't want answers. She wanted this dietary permission slip: *Please excuse Cathy from making nutrition-related changes in her life. She's incorrigible, and nothing will ever work.*

Cathy wanted validation of her perceived failure. She wanted me to realize she was different from *everyone else* (the group of people with which she has nothing in common).

Cathy wanted to believe that everyone else controls personal eating habits. Everyone else's lifestyle changes come easily and effortlessly. These beliefs gave Cathy permission to stay just the way she was.

Setting yourself apart from the world is often a reflection of your resistance to change.

Changes *are* difficult. Making changes to my own eating habits continues to challenge me. This point bugged Cathy, too. She wanted to shock me with her failings. She wanted me to say, "You ate an entire bar of chocolate when you intended to eat one square? Unbelievable!" or "You ate nothing at the wedding reception but later scarfed down the cake you saved for your kids? I never!"

I can't say "I never" because I have. Cathy can't "out sin" me. I've done it all myself. My successes and failures are no better or worse than anyone else's; they're just different. That's annoying to someone who wants permission to *not* be like everyone else. Darn.

Here's a tip: The best thing about failure is the opportunity to try something else the next time. Lifestyle changes may seem difficult, but there are infinite ways to go about making them.

Muscles need exercise to develop, so why wouldn't developing the palate be the same way? Eating better doesn't happen overnight. It takes training to develop a taste for healthier fare.

When you hit on a successful behavior, repeat it for at least thirty days in a row to make it a habit. Some need longer periods of reinforcement, others less. Redirect the inner chatter that says, "Oh well, I blew it. I may as well finish the whole cake." Think of your *next bite* as an opportunity to get back on track. Instead of putting off improvements to tomorrow, next week, or next year, think in immediate time frames.

A wise friend of mine says, "Failure is a great place to make a U-turn." Maybe I'll invite her to lunch with Cathy.

OFF LABEL – I DARE YOU

It was a big deal when the first "official" fibromyalgia pharmaceutical drug hit the market. You may not be aware, but before, all drugs prescribed specifically for fibromyalgia were considered "off label." That means drugs labeled for conditions other than the one treated.

Labeling is vital to drug companies. It speeds up the insurance process, and provides doctors with an established treatment protocol. It's like a pre-packaged cake mix. Necessary ingredients are grouped together for ease and simplicity. Pluck the box from the shelf and you're assured success. Likewise, your diagnosis comes with a pre-set mix of recommended drugs and treatments.

There are, however, detriments to labeling. Labeling leads to stereotypes that are restrictive, confining, limiting. Fibrofolk have preconceived ideas about themselves and others. This is the dangerous one-size-fits-all paradigm. If chronic illness proves anything, it's that we're *not* all alike. For one, pain is a primary symptom; for another, it could be fatigue or fogginess. Successful treatment varies as much as the symptoms.

I choose to live off label. Some of my activities fit with the "typical fibro-person," but others don't. I'm often asked, "Can you do that?" when I mention weightlifting, fitness classes, or even backyard games. Of course I can!

I make my own definition of who I am and what I'm capable of. I suggest the same for you. Go ahead. Remove the label of fibromyalgia (or chronic fatigue, etc.). Remove the stigma. Live your own life; find your own solutions and, most of all, make your own rules.

I dare you.

WORDS – WORTH

I'm a word person. I love words and phrases as much as a chef loves herbs and spices. I savor the sound and feel of them as they dangle from fingertips hovering over the keyboard. One of my favorite words is "abide." So much depth and meaning for one itty-bitty, barely multi-syllabic word.

When something abides with you, you not only know it in your mind and feel it in your heart; it lives and breathes in you. That's why abide is often used in context with faith. If faith were simply a lesson to learn, we'd cram like crazy and take the final. Over and done. Instead, faith is a living, breathing entity. It changes; it expands and contracts with the elements of time and experience.

My desire for wellness abides with me daily. My methods are constantly changing and evolving. It's not just stuff I know in my head and feel in my heart.

Wellness lives within me.

I know a pastor who made a tough decision. He uprooted his family and swapped a secure city church for an obscure rural one. An unpopular decision, it was a risky move that took courage and serious skin-thickening.

It's not a surprise that this man has settled into his new life with vigor. He's found what he sought, though he was unable to define it before the move. He's a changed man, fulfilled. Even better, he's healthy.

You see, before the move he ran around caring for everyone else. He neglected his own needs. He's a bright guy so he knew he lacked balance. He attempted change by spiffing up his diet and adding exercise to his routine. It didn't "take."

Now that he's living like Daniel Boone (sans shotgun and coonskin cap), he's found a health regimen that works for him.

His weight loss is significant, but more important, he's well. His balanced lifestyle is apparent to all.

In the search for wellness, weight loss is not the ultimate destination. People often visualize their ideal weight goal as a big X on a treasure map. But if they do, they're missing the point. Weight is only one component of your health journey. Personal change must be your travel companion.

Wellness arrives when you find that place you can call "home." Not a tangible home, but a path that feels right. A path paved by self-discovery, curiosity, and an open mind. That's where the seed of faith begins, and wellness abides.

HELLO, IT'S SO NICE TO MEET ME

For umpteen pages now, I've illustrated ways in which my health has improved. I've been transformed by the education my illness has provided. In reviewing my health history, I feel a strange "set apart" feeling from the person I used to be. I barely recognize her.

Shouldn't we at least understand the person who stares back at us in the mirror? This thought isn't new; Socrates said, "The unexamined life is not worth living."

Self-examination plus action equals success. With the lifestyle changes I've made, I've succeeded in improving these areas: pain, fatigue, digestion, sleep patterns, physical strength, energy, balance, posture, memory, vision, mood, weight, skin condition (bruising, blotches, dry, etc.), hair, natural immunity (resistance to colds, flu, etc.) and reduced numbness/tingling in my extremities.

It's with great irony that I recognize another fact: I no longer care about the name of my condition. For so long, I placed one foot in front of the other in focused pursuit of a name, a diagnosis. My arrival at that name was to be the end of my race. Of course, when I got there, I found no finish line; it was just the starter's gate for yet another race.

I, like many, have a multitude of conditions. Does one name really fit? Something like *FibroChronicAdrenalColitisHormonal-ExhaustedSleeplessMindBogglingSyndrome* may be more accurate, but tough to write on insurance forms. Perhaps *Systems Gone Berserk Syndrome* says it all.

Each of us is as different as our constellations of symptoms. The causes of our illnesses are different, and the remedies needed are different. Using one identifier to label our conditions is like identifying individual stars as the Milky Way.

So why the kerfuffle about a name? If the name of my condition changed today, I wouldn't care. It matters little. What does matter is that I've learned how I "broke" my system and how I can "fix" it.

It's no coincidence that taking charge of my health led me to a better place, physically and emotionally. I've stated the causes of my health issues and the solutions I've found … so far.

Self-examination is an ongoing process. I look forward to a lifetime of discoveries. When I began this journey, I blamed many causes of my illness on my nature as a stubborn Midwestern Norwegian. Ironically, those same traits have helped me pave the way toward rebuilding wellness.

Now, isn't it time for another cup of tea?

"Life consists not simply in what heredity and environment do to us, but in what we make out of what they do to us."

—Thomas Dekker

Chapter 9

On your mark, get set—KNOW!

The ten root causes of chronic illness are summarized here. Further details on each of these subjects can be found in books, videos, and websites listed in the Resources section of this book. Abundant sources are available to help determine the impact these root causes have on your personal health concerns.

৶

My husband has a theory he calls "the nut behind the button." After decades of working in the garage door industry, he learned that many operational failures were not related to the equipment at all. Rather, the failure was likely the person (nut) pushing the opening device (button).

Oftentimes, dismantled equipment, electrical breaker failures, or missing batteries were to blame. Many an embarrassed homeowner uttered an apology when a service technician found a power cord plugged into a guitar amp instead of a garage door opener.

In the same way, health problems provide you with a "nut behind the button" opportunity. Have you tracked your illness to the source? Have you attempted to fix the symptoms without unearthing the cause?

As Ricky often told Lucy, "You've got some 'splainin' to do." Health solutions begin with a little 'splainin'.

We must understand the root causes before applying the "cure."

TEN ROOTS TO A BETTER YOU

It's logical to look for someone or something to blame for your sickness. We all do it. It's easy to point the finger at doctors or treatments that failed, but is that fair? The foundations of health are complicated.

Chronic illness results from contributing co-factors. No single criterion creates disease ("disease" meaning, lack of wellness). A combination of factors, or a "perfect storm" scenario, compromises health. Not all of these factors must be present to create illness, but it is likely to have several, many of which overlap.

These ten root causes play a role in the development of chronic illness:

1.   Genetic Predisposition
2.   Physical Injury or Trauma
3.   Emotional Trauma
4.   Malnourishment
5.   External Toxins
6.   Internal Toxins
7.   Inflammation
8.   Infection
9.   Hormonal Imbalance
10. Thyroid Dysfunction

A brief discussion of each follows.

1) Genetic Predisposition

We're all born with a predisposition to some health conditions. Our genetic makeup follows our parents' and that of generations past. Conditions such as cancers, diabetes, and autoimmune illnesses can be traced through our lineage. Genetic history, as a diagnostic tool, can help point doctors in the right direction.

A genetic predisposition is no guarantee of illness. If your mother has rheumatoid arthritis, it does not mean you or your children will have that or any other autoimmune-related condition. It's simply one factor in your genetic makeup.

Genetic predisposition does not leave you helpless. You're not a slave to your genes. Does heart disease run in your family? Forewarned is forearmed. Your lifestyle choices (dietary choices in particular) have a great influence over correcting and mitigating genetic tendencies.

2) Physical Injury or Trauma

A car accident is an obvious source of physical trauma. Other accidents may lead to broken bones, cuts, and bruises; but what about less obvious sources of injury? Perhaps you had a lengthy bout of pneumonia as a child or a lingering illness. Physical traumas at any age can compromise health.

Some traumas, such as surgeries, aren't accidental, but are no less harmful. Medications required for surgery (including anesthesia) can be very traumatic to the body. Of course, the incision itself is traumatic, too. Healing from surgery may take months or years. Surgery traumas are often paired with emotional traumas: accidents, distressful medical diagnoses, and losses such as limbs, organs, or even a child.

3) Emotional Traumas

It's common to find that people dealing with fibromyalgia, chronic fatigue, and/or autoimmune conditions have experienced one or more serious emotional traumas. These strategic events are so impactful that the body goes into shock. While the event is emotional in nature, it's severe enough to cause physical manifestations.

I think of these extreme traumatic events as "emotional earthquakes." Oftentimes, they occur in childhood, and denial of their existence takes a toll. Emotional traumas keep the body suspended in a state of inner anxiety (which may contribute to post-traumatic stress disorder). Negative thoughts are a source of continuous trauma. The body is unable to heal fully until the anxiety is resolved.

Stress in general is a common denominator for people suffering from chronic illness. Stress tears at the fabric of the immune and hormonal systems. Understanding how to manage stress is *not* optional. Everyone experiences stress, but not everyone deals well with it. Call them coping mechanisms or learned skills — stress management methods are necessary to healing.

4) Malnourishment

Nothing "lights my fire" more than a rousing conversation about nutrition. I've become a nutritional evangelist, counseling anyone who'll listen about unhealthy eating habits. I'd probably throw a body block in front of a toddler if his parents attempted to give him a baby bottle filled with soda.

Don't underestimate the role that nutrition plays in your wellness plan. It's the foundation of health — where good (or bad) health begins.

The effects of poor nutrition may go unnoticed for a time, but discovering the deterioration caused by nutritional deficiencies is an ugly find. Malnourishment compromises your bones, muscles, and organs. Nutritional deficiencies are a primary cause of many chronic illnesses, with other root causes as co-factors.

5) External Toxins

Thinking of environmental toxins (or, more accurately, toxicants/toxics) typically brings pesticides and herbicides to mind. After further thought, products such as paints, solvents, lacquers, dyes, etc., may be added to the list.

But what of the toxic products used *inside* your home — many used daily? Cleaning, laundry, and air-freshening products often contain harmful, toxic ingredients. Some products intended for direct skin contact — such as fragrances, antiperspirants, hair care products, and cosmetics — contain toxins as well.

Look also to your surroundings. Environmental toxins may exist in your home or workplace from molds, gasses emitted from treated lumber, carpet backings, and chemically-treated fabrics.

Some external toxins (pesticides and herbicides) can become internal ones when contaminated fruits and vegetables are eaten.

6) Internal Toxins

Foods with harmful additives and preservatives may prove toxic as might pharmaceuticals (including over the counter [OTC] medications), internal foreign objects such as implants, and heavy metals (internalized via contaminated foods, vaccines, and dental amalgams).

The liver and kidneys (filtering organs) become overworked as they attempt to filter ingested chemicals and toxins. Symptoms of an overburdened liver include fatigue, exhaustion, weakness, easy bruising of the skin, abdominal pain, and nausea.

While not all food additives and preservatives are toxic, it's a good idea to review lists available from consumer safety sources such as The Center for Science in the Public Interest, http://www.cspinet.org/.

7) Inflammation

An inflamed body is one under siege; it's the body's attempt at healing. Intestinal inflammation stems from improper digestion of processed foods and from foods that cause an allergic response. Foods that don't "agree" with you are guilty of causing an allergic response whether you're truly allergic or intolerant.

Diets high in sugary and processed foods and some pharmaceuticals (mainly antibiotics) disrupt the balance of intestinal flora in the digestive tract. This leads to an acid/alkaline imbalance, allowing yeast or candida to proliferate.

Inflammation in the digestive tract causes malabsorption of nutrients and a compromised immune system, among other factors.

Muscles, joints, and body tissues are also susceptible to inflammation — a primary source of pain.

8) Infection

There's a long-standing theory that autoimmune illnesses are triggered by infection. Links between viruses and chronic conditions have been documented. Many chronically-ill people claim their symptoms first began after an illness such as mononucleosis or a lingering undiagnosed viral infection.

Combined with heredity and nutritional deficiencies, infection is a likely co-factor in the cause of many autoimmune conditions.

Viruses can remain dormant for long periods. This blurs the correlation between infection and the onset of illness. Some people are symptomatic right away, others, years or even decades later.

In the case of Lyme disease and/or borreliosis, etc., the infection left behind from a tick bite triggers a constellation of autoimmune symptoms. A diagnosis of fibromyalgia, chronic fatigue, rheumatoid arthritis, lupus, multiple sclerosis, etc., may address symptoms, but leaves the underlying cause untreated. Both the infection and the damages caused by tick-related infection must be addressed.

9) Hormonal Imbalance

Hormonal imbalances can be a source of many dysfunctions in the body. Hormones affect the metabolism, immune system, and also sex drive, moods, and emotions. Symptoms similar to allergies and hay fever can be attributed to hormonal imbalances.

For women, hormonal imbalances wreak havoc in additional ways. PMS (premenstrual syndrome), fibroids, anxiety, hair loss, foggy thinking, headaches/migraines, weight gain (water retention), osteoporosis, endometriosis, and wrinkled skin are symptomatic of hormonal dysfunction.

The strong connection between hormone imbalance and fibromyalgia is a significant factor in why more women than men are affected by this condition.

10) Thyroid Dysfunction

Low thyroid function can be blamed for many symptoms including sleep disturbances, metabolism impact (resulting in weight gain), mood swings, intolerance to cold temperatures, and brittle hair and nails.

It's important to note that many fibrofolk exhibit symptoms consistent with thyroid dysfunction, yet their typical doctor's visit blood tests reflect "normal" results. The standard normal ranges for testing may not catch low-functioning thyroids, leaving patients in the lurch.

It's likely that untreated low thyroid function is common among fibrofolk and others dealing with autoimmune-related illnesses.

TIME TO PONDER

How many of the above causes do you believe apply to you? I'd guess some may be more familiar than you'd like. Other than genetics, there's no right or wrong combination of the remaining causes. Each person is different; each illness is different.

Identifying the causes of chronic illness is the first step toward correcting them. Address the individual problems, paying close attention to how they relate to one another. Many, such as hormone and thyroid function, are linked. One root cause cannot be addressed without the others.

For example, what if your home were built on a toxic-waste dump? You could "eat clean" and take the finest supplements but never completely "fix" your health issues without addressing your environment.

Underlying health problems are not typically as obvious as

living on a trash heap, so consider each root cause to pinpoint the sources of *your* health concerns.

৶৯

Now that you know what's at the root of your illness, it's time to put that knowledge into action. Health maintenance isn't a one-shot deal; it's more like perpetual motion. Would you do a lube and tune to your car just once? Health maintenance and the motivation to move forward are ongoing, continuous lifestyle changes.

> "*Dig where the gold is, unless you just need some exercise.*"
>
> —John M. Capozzi

When dealing with a health crisis, many people arrive at desperation. Good, that's a great place to be! It's the "I'll try anything" type of desperation that leads to an open mind. It's the perfect time to start a new regimen, a new plan for healthy living. Once you've achieved better health, remember to keep moving. There's no finish line to cross.

At one point, I thought I "beat" fibromyalgia; I was symptom-free for more than a year. I became over-confident and slacked off from my healthy habits. I nibbled on junk food, failed to replace some supplements as they ran out. I skipped going to the gym here and there. Big deal, right? But when big-time stress arrived, I spiraled smack-dab back to the beginning.

I'm not the only one. I've seen others begin a "get healthy" kick, get well, and then forget why they did it in the first place. I call this "get well amnesia."

When you revert to former habits, don't be surprised when your good health reverts, too.

৶৯

I hope that you now recognize these overarching themes in healing: self-awareness, tenacity, and self-respect.

You must devise a plan of action, take action, and monitor how the action works for you — and only you. The symptoms of chronic illness differ for each of us, as do the remedies.

I've found dramatic physical and emotional healing through

the methods spelled out in this book, and it's my hope that others will find success, too. But my path will not be the same as anyone else's. The root causes of my chronic illness are not identical to anyone's and neither are the remedies. It's common for frustrated people to grasp at both successes *and* failures. Successes, because they learned something new; failures, because they confirmed something they *believe* they already knew.

It's time to focus on the successes; above all, don't *expect* failures.

Of all the hints and suggestions in this book, it's likely that one or two will strike a nerve or rub you the wrong way. If you disagree with a finer point, don't let that detract from your goal. Developing a case of Baby With the Bathwater Syndrome leads some to discount important healing ideas simply because of a disagreement with one or more of the components.

I once heard a seminar attendee say it was pointless to listen to my speech because I mentioned bell peppers. "Everyone knows," she said, "that we [meaning fibrofolk] can't eat nightshade vegetables."

It's true that some people with inflammatory conditions benefit from the elimination of nightshade vegetables from their diets. However, throwing out my entire speech on nutrition, digestion, and metabolism simply because I eat bell peppers is representative of Baby With the Bathwater Syndrome. (NOTE: I have experimented with eliminating nightshade vegetables from my diet and have found no adverse effect from bell peppers.)

> "*Honest differences are often a healthy sign of progress.*"
>
> —Mahatma Gandhi

If an exercise I've recommended doesn't work for you, don't conclude physical fitness isn't your thing. If you find my reference to animal proteins annoying because you're a vegan, look beyond the minutia and grasp the big picture.

When it comes to making changes, as long as you move toward *healthier living*, you'll move toward *healing*.

Keep learning. Keep trying. You'll soon discover that right after tenacity kicks in, self-respect follows.

RECIPES FOR SUCCESS

What do you carry in your Basket of Well? Each nutritional tidbit, exercise know-how, or stress-relieving tool propels your personal healing journey forward. It's not about finding *the* singular method; it's about accumulating a variety of them to suit your individual needs. While I don't have all the answers, I do have an increased awareness of my condition and of what I can do to help myself get better.

Here's a select few of my favorites. Stir them into your own personal health recipes and test them for success.

Eating –
>   *Keep it light — keep it bright*
>   (low-calorie veggies in lots of healthful colors)
>
>   *Foods to ban — from bag, box, or can*
>   (choose whole foods, avoid artificial ingredients)
>
>   *Foods that fuel — foods that fool*
>   (choose nutrient-dense foods, no trans fats, HFCS, artificial sweeteners, MSG, etc.)

Exercise –
>   *Use your brain to train*
>   (choose exercises for both mind *and* body)
>
>   *Don't let a blip tip the scales*
>   (weigh in regularly to stay on track)
>
>   *Slacker — snacker*
>   (regular exercise helps stave off mindless eating)

Stress Relief –
>   *Eeyeore no more*
>   (focus on the positive)
>
>   *Choose to lose*
>   (decide to drop unhealthy habits, thoughts, behaviors)
>
>   *Mind finds*
>   (pray and/or meditate regularly)

SUE'S INCOMPLETE LIST OF "MIRACLE" SOLUTIONS

Solutions to the chronic illness puzzle are ever-changing. New remedies appear on the horizon as fast as outdated ones disappear. Though I've tried a great many of these solutions, I don't have personal experience with all of them, and, therefore, cannot attest to their miraculous properties. The point is, solutions (miracle or not) can be found in traditional and non-traditional therapies.

This list is by no means exhaustive.

- Acupuncture/acupressure
- Apple cider vinegar
- Aqua aerobics / hydrotherapy (in non-chlorinated water)
- Auriculotherapy
- Ayurveda healing
- Belly dancing
- Biofeedback
- Chiropractic
- Colon, liver, and/or kidney cleanse
- Compounded natural hormones/supplements
- CoQ10
- Cranial electrotherapy stimulation
- Dance/creative movement therapy
- Deep breathing
- Detoxing (including elimination of heavy metals)
- D-ribose
- Drink more water (and/or alkaline water)
- Emu oil, topically
- Energy therapy
- Essential minerals
- Essential oils, topically
- Exercise/fitness training
- Far-infrared saunas
- Fish/krill oil
- Floss your teeth (good dental hygiene)
- Gin raisins
- Guaifenesin
- Holistic infusion treatments
- Hypnosis
- Increased dietary fiber (from plant-based, natural sources)
- Infrared light therapy

- Iodine
- Laser therapy
- Magnets
- Massage therapy
- Mattress/Bedding (healing materials such as foam, down, wool)
- Natural sunlight exposure (vitamin D)
- Nightshade vegetable elimination
- Oil pulling (an oral cleansing treatment)
- Pet therapy
- Physical therapy
- Pilates
- Prayer/Meditation/ MTT
- Probiotics and Digestive enzymes
- Raw food diets
- Reflexology
- Reiki and feldenkreis therapies
- Resveratrol
- Skin brushing (for improved circulation)
- Sleep (and good sleep hygiene)
- Slow food movement
- Sound healing/therapy (vibrational healing)
- Spirulina/chlorella
- Stretching
- Super-nutrient berries and berry juices
- Sweat lodges
- Tai chi/ Qigong
- Transcutaneous electrical nerve stimulation (TeNS)
- Trigger point therapy
- Turbosonic therapy
- Vegetable (raw) juicing
- Virgin coconut oil and raw coconut products
- Whole body vibration (WBV)
- Yoga (restorative)

RELATIVE HEREDITY

Some say that chronic illness is like a closed door or a roadblock to progress. I think it's more like a mirror reflecting who we are as "sick" people and how that came to be. Chronic illness gives us ample opportunities to refine our abilities, ingenuity, and resolve.

Once we've examined our reflections, the path we take is up to us. Coming full circle, I kicked my Midwestern upbringing into

> "*What lies behind us and what lies before us are small matters compared to what lies within us.*"
>
> —Ralph Waldo Emerson

high gear — learned to work within my strengths. I chose to replace habits that were no longer working for me with ones healthier and, ultimately, more fulfilling.

I'd even say, if I had it to do over again, I'd do things the same way (perhaps without the *three* swine flu vaccinations I received in the seventies). I'd choose to take my lumps as they came, knowing they provided priceless education.

I did the best I could with what I knew then and put into practice what I know now. Isn't that all that anyone can ask?

Inside, I'm still just a kid from Iowa. The long-reaching roots of my heritage still touch me from two thousand miles away. I grew up with the beliefs that I should respect my elders, never giggle in church, treat my community as I would my hometown, and always serve Velveeta® cheese when company comes to dinner.

Well, two out of four isn't bad, is it?

"*Health is a state of complete physical, mental, and social well-being, and not merely the absence of disease or infirmity.*"

—World Health Organization, 1948

Glossary

Alkaline water/ionized water. Water filtered through specialized equipment that ionizes minerals to change the pH levels and create alkaline water.

Applied kinesiology. A form of muscle response testing that uses the body's electrical system to identify systemic and nutritional deficiencies; also used to identify and eliminate allergies, release emotional issues, and strengthen body systems; typically used by natural health practitioners and chiropractors.

Artificial sweeteners. Aspartame (NutraSweet, Equal), Sucralose (Splenda), Saccharin (Sweet & Low, Sugar Twin).

BFF. Best friend forever; contemporary lingo often used in text messages.

BHT/BHA/Benzoic acid. Chemicals used as food preservatives.

Candida / Candidiasis. Systemic yeast/fungal overgrowth (yeast infection) typically affecting immunocompromised individuals.

Carbohydrates. Organic compound that serves as a major source of energy. There are both "good" and "bad" carbohydrates. Foods that contain the highest amount of carbohydrates are starchy foods such as breads, pastas, potatoes, and cereals. Plant-based, high- fiber carbohydrates (vegetables/fruits) are a vital part of a healthy diet.

Costochondritis. A condition defined by tenderness (pain) in the upper breastbone or lower ribs. Caused by inflammation of the cartilage that attaches the ribs to the breastbone. Pain may be more severe when sitting or reclining. Acute pain may lead some patients to feel as if they're having a heart attack.

Cox-2 inhibitors. A class of nonsteroidal, anti-inflammatory medications including Vioxx, Celebrex, and Bextra.

DDT. A contact insecticide spray used extensively in the agriculture industry from the 1940s through the early 1970s.

Digestive enzymes. Natural enzymes that assist food digestion. Because of over-processed food sources, it's increasingly necessary to supplement the standard American diet with over-the-counter digestive enzymes, which can be found in most health food stores.

Digestive system. Includes the mouth, digestive tract, and other organs that help to break down, digest and absorb foods, and eliminate wastes.

Fartlek. Swedish term meaning *speed variation*; most commonly refers to athletic interval training.

Fibrofolk. Those diagnosed with fibromyalgia and other related autoimmune conditions.

Functional medicine. Healing field of professionals that focuses on the sources or causes of illness rather than on the symptoms.

GERD. Gastroesophageal reflux disease; a condition where food or liquids reverses from the stomach up to the esophagus, causing irritation and heartburn. Changes in diet may eliminate this condition by naturally reducing stomach acids.

GI. Glycemic index; ranks the effects of carbohydrates in foods on blood sugar levels; especially helpful information for maintaining a healthy metabolism and for people dealing with diabetes. Glycemic index and glycemic load tables, including a comprehensive list of common American foods, can be found at http://www.mendosa.com/common_foods.htm.

GL. Glycemic load; adds the component of portion size to the glycemic index; provides a more detailed resource measuring the impact a food has on blood sugar levels. Glycemic index and glycemic load tables, including a comprehensive list of common American foods, can be found at http://www.mendosa.com/common_foods.htm.

HFCS. High fructose corn syrup; a processed food starch that can be found in sodas, salad dressings, granola bars, and in many processed foods. The rise of obesity statistics in the United States are often reported in tandem with the rise of HFCS use.

IBS. Irritable bowel syndrome; condition where the lower intestinal tract becomes inflamed and fails to function properly. Constipation, gassiness, bloating, diarrhea, and painful cramping are all symptoms of IBS. Relief may be found through dietary adjustments and stress-relieving activities.

Ischemia. Restricted blood flow (and oxygen) affecting the body. Cardiac ischemia is a condition demonstrating restricted blood flow to the heart.

Kübler-Ross model. The five stages of grief as introduced by psychiatrist Elisabeth Kübler-Ross in 1969. 1) denial, 2) anger, 3) bargaining, 4) depression, and 5) acceptance. Grief may move back and forth between these stages, not necessarily in a sequential manner.

Leaky gut syndrome. A condition where the walls of the bowel become damaged. The gut becomes porous, and therefore leaks; possible causes include antibiotics, inflammation, food sensitivities or allergies, parasites, poor diet, and/or infections.

MFA. Master's degree in fine arts.

MTT. Meridian tapping technique; a method of tapping on specific acupressure points to facilitate physical and emotional healing.

Metabolic or nutritional typing. The science of customizing a person's diet based on his or her personal metabolism.

Nutrigenetics. *See Nutrigenomics.*

Nutrigenomics. The study of the effects of foods on a person's genetics. Tailor-made dietary recommendations for individuals based on genetic makeup rather than on the general population.

Neurotransmitters. Chemicals that transmit signals from one neuron to the next. Neurotransmitters perform a vital function as communicators in the body.

Nightshade vegetables. Generally considered to include tomatoes, potatoes, peppers, eggplant, ground cherries, gooseberries, goji berries (wolfberries), and tobacco. (NOTE: Foods documented as nightshade vegetables vary widely depending on the source.)

Normals. All other folk than fibrofolk; those not having fibromyalgia and/or overlapping autoimmune conditions.

OTC. Over the counter medications available for purchase at drugstores or retailers as opposed to medications available only by prescription.

Omega-3s. The naturally occurring fatty acids found in many fish oils (krill, herring, tuna, sardines, salmon, mackerel, sturgeon, anchovies), some vegetables, seeds, and nuts. Some of the many benefits of omega-3s are reduced pain/swelling from rheumatoid conditions, improved cognitive functions (used for Alzheimer's disease, depression, Attention Deficit Hyperactivity Disorder), healthier skin, and reduced risk of heart disease.

Organic. Produce grown without pesticides or herbicides. Organic animal products generally raised free range, without added hormones or antibiotics. Non GMO (Genetically Modified Organism) foods.

PBS. Public broadcast system; public television is a source of free educational programming on a wide variety of subjects.

PTSD. Post-traumatic stress disorder. An anxiety disorder triggered by a traumatic event. While PTSD is known as an emotional disorder, the effects are both physical and emotional. PTSD effects may linger for years or decades if unaddressed and left untreated.

Probiotics. Supplements of live microorganisms taken to improve digestion. Intestinal flora become unbalanced through improper diet and frequent use of pharmaceuticals such as antibiotics. Supplementation of probiotics has been linked to improved microbial balance, better digestive health, and lower candida overgrowth.

Qigong. A form of martial arts defined by slow, meditative movements and controlled breathing. Qigong is reported to have healing effects on the body, including reduced pain and improved circulation, immune system, and memory.

REM. Rapid eye movement. Refers to the deepest stage of sleep during which the most restorative health benefits are achieved; dreams most often occur in the REM stage of sleep.

Satiety. The feeling of satisfaction after eating, the absence of hunger. Foods that are typically slower to digest give a greater feeling of satiety such as fiber-rich veggies and proteins. Adding fiber to your diet is a healthy and effective way to curb hunger.

Saturated/Unsaturated fats. Saturated fats are typically solid at room temperature. These include meat fats, cream, butter, and cheese fats. Unsaturated fats remain liquid at room temperature and are obtained from fish (krill, herring, tuna, sardines, salmon, mackerel, sturgeon, anchovies), vegetables, nuts, or seeds. Some unsaturated fats provide a valuable source of omega-3s, which are an essential part of a healthy diet.

Serotonin. A neurotransmitter generated primarily in the digestive tract; known to help regulate mood, sleep, muscle contraction, memory, and appetite.

Sleep hygiene. Habits and rituals followed to ensure proper sleep. May include relaxation methods before bed, consistent sleep (and waking) times, and setting standard room temperature and darkness levels.

Stevia. Whole-leaf stevia is a natural, plant-based sweetener available in a variety of liquid or powdered forms from most holistic or health food stores.

Substance P. A neurotransmitter that triggers the sensation of pain (as well as some other related functions). An overabundance of substance P has been found in patients diagnosed with fibromyalgia and other chronic pain conditions.

Titer. The measurement of a substance in a solution. An antibody titer defines the concentration or level of antibodies in the blood.

Toxins. Substances known to be poisonous. Those formed by man-made substances are technically known as *toxicants.*

Trans fats. Partially hydrogenated oils (PHOs). Man-made fats that are engineered to have a long shelf life. Typically used in mass-produced bakery items, snack foods, and in fried foods for fast food restaurants.

Vetted. Appraised information, verification of accuracy.

Villi. Small, finger-like hairs lining the intestinal walls. Good villi health is critical to nutrient absorption and food digestion.

Whole foods. Foods derived as close to their source as possible; foods not processed or altered from their natural state. Eating whole foods rather than processed foods is often referred to as *eating clean.*

Resources

GENERAL HEALTH WEBSITES

http://www.mercola.com/
Dr. Joseph Mercola, author; newsletter, searchable health news
database, books, products

http://www.drhyman.com/, http://www.ultrametabolism.com/
Dr. Mark Hyman, author; medical advice focusing on metabolism,
weight loss, and brain functions, books

http://www.treatingandbeating.com/
Dr. Rodger Murphree, author; nutritional counseling specialized
for fibromyalgia and autoimmune conditions, books, products

http://www.knowthecause.com/
Doug Kaufmann, author, TV program host; research articles,
books, product recommendations, links to syndicated programs

http://www.drcolbert.com/
Dr. Don Colbert, author; books, supplements, articles

http://www.prohealth.com/
Research news, newsletter, articles, supplements, support communities

http://www.six-wise.com/
Articles, newsletter, comprehensive holistic living resource

http://www.myhealthybalance.com/ and http://www.ichange.com/
Linda Miner, RNC, nutritional expert; blogs, articles, TV programs,
personal nutritional assessments, weight loss counseling

http://www.goodworkswellness.com/
Pamela Reilly, speaker, Naturopath, Raw Foods Life Coach; blog, articles

http://www.functionalmedicine.org/
The Institute for Functional Medicine (includes directory of
functional medicine practitioners)

FIBROMYALGIA AND CHRONIC ILLNESS SUPPORT WEBSITES AND BLOGS:

http://www.butyoudontlooksick.com/
Message boards, chat room, [source of popular "Spoon Theory"
helpful to explain energy levels to "normals"], articles, craft/
cooking ideas, gift shop

http://www.fmaware.org/
National Fibromyalgia Association website providing information,
resources, education, online magazine, doctor referral listings

http://www.workingwithchronicillness.com/
Book, website, and blog encouraging women with autoimmune
conditions to work and remain active.

http://www.wellwire.com/
Holistic community, advice from naturopathic providers and variety
of guest writers

http://fibrohaven.wordpress.com/
Dannette Rusnak; informational fibromyalgia blog, news,
research articles

http://www.thecanaryreport.com/
Forum to educate and unite people with multiple chemical
sensitivities, blog, chat room, photos, resources

http://www.glutenfreefox.com/
"World's Gluten-Free Search Engine," articles, expert resources,
food listings, skin care resources gluten-free food suggestions
for pets

http://www.invisibleillnessweek.com/
Blog, articles, ideas, gifts, inspiration, information on an annual week-long conference including speakers, seminars, online events

http://www.chronicbabe.com/
Online community of young women living with chronic illness

SUPPLEMENTS AND HEALTHY LIVING PRODUCT WEBSITES:

http://www.attractingabundance.com/
Carol Look; Meridian Tapping Technique resources

http://www.shopnutritionplus.com/
Diane Wendell, ND, CNM, nutritionist; wellness center, articles, resources, products

http://www.tropicaltraditions.com/
Virgin coconut products, green nutrients, organic meats, recipes, articles, various holistic and organic specialties

http://www.suzannes.com/
Holistic online store, supplements, vitamins, homeopathy remedies

http://www.bestlifedesign.com/
Dr. Mollie Marti, author, speaker, life coach; articles, resources on wellness, finances, healthy living topics

http://www.freshfocusskincare.com/
Holistic, all-natural, plant-based skin care, makeup products, non-imported handbags, accessories

http://www.shoporganic.com/
Organic products, foods, vitamins, household products, pet supplies

http://www.arbonne.com/
Botanical skin care, makeup, nutritional supplement products

EXERCISE AND HEALTHY MOVEMENT WEBSITES:

http://www.t-tapp.com/
Teresa Tapp's books, exercise and fitness DVDs, articles, products

http://www.thegroveapproach.com/
Karen Groves' yoga for fibromyalgia DVDs, including Fibroga®, fitness products

http://www.nubalance.com/
Melissa Stewart's tai chi DVD, alkaline water equipment sales and information, nutritional supplement products

BOOKS:

Dr. Mercola's Total Health Program: The Proven Plan to Prevent Disease and Premature Aging, Optimize Weight and Live Longer by Dr. Joseph Mercola; Mercola.com; 2004.
A comprehensive health guide including information on nutrition, disease prevention, weight management, and recipes.

The Ultra Simple Diet: Kick-Start Your Metabolism and Safely Lose Up to 10 Pounds in 7 Days by Dr. Mark Hyman; Pocket Books; 2007.
A weight-loss handbook explaining metabolism, meal planning, and fitness for the chronically ill patient.

The Bible Cure for Candida and Yeast Infections by Dr. Don Colbert; Siloam Press division of Strang Communications Company; 2001.
A guide explaining the origins of and natural solutions for yeast/candida overgrowth. Includes a simple questionnaire and food lists.

Mariel's Kitchen: Simple Ingredients for a Delicious and Satisfying Life by Mariel Hemingway; HarperCollins; 2009.
A cookbook that goes far beyond the kitchen. Includes recipes and lifestyle hints enhanced with gorgeous, full-color photographs.

The Maker's Diet by Jordan Rubin; Berkley Books; 2005.

The true story of Jordan Rubin detailing his desperate search for health. His success story includes food plans and recipes.

The First 30 Days: Your Guide to Making Any Change Easier by Ariane de Bonvoisin; HarperCollins; 2008.
A powerful teaching book that describes how to make the tough decisions that bring on positive, life-altering change.

The Ultimate Weight Solution Food Guide by Dr. Phil McGraw; Pocket Books; 2004.
Food guide providing charts of calorie and nutrient counts for many natural, pre-packaged, and restaurant foods.

Fabulous Food Detectives by Susan E. Ingebretson; Playbooks, Inc.; 2008.
An educational book on nutrition and deciphering food labels written for children in a reader's theater format. Available through Playbook's® catalog of books. Search http://www.playbooks.com/, under Stories by Topic/Theme, and then Health/Nutrition.

DVDs:

Food Matters, http://www.foodmatters.tv/

Sweet Misery: A Poisoned World, http://www.amazon.com/, http://www.mercola.com/, other health-related sources, (artificial sweetener documentary)

Living with Fibromyalgia: A Journey of Hope and Understanding, http://www.livingwithfm.com/

Try It On Everything: Discover the Power of EFT®, http://www.thetappingsolution.com/

I Can Make You Thin, http://www.mckenna.com/, (Paul McKenna's tapping methods, self-hypnosis, affirmations)

Acknowledgements

Many thanks to my family for their love and support during my journey from chronic illness to chronic wellness. I especially thank my hubby and pup for being there when I needed them most. I'd also like to thank Mari Lou, Barb, Adam, Pat, Marly, Cindy, Jennifer, and Susan for their assistance and encouragement.

Index

A

G

H

L

Labels
    Nutrition   50, 54-56, 66
    Pharmaceutical   151-152
    Products/health and beauty   34, 142, 144
Laser therapy
    Miracle solution   167
Leaky gut syndrome   60, 173
Leptin
    Appetite control   63-65
Liver   11
    Cleanse, miracle solution   166
    Toxins   160
Lupus   15, 134
    Autoimmune   22
    Lyme disease, infection   161
    Identifying with   114
Lyme disease   15
    Infection   161

M

Magnets
    Miracle solution   167
Malnourish   11
    A root cause of chronic illness   158, 159–160
    Intestinal health   52
    Symptom of chronic illness   16
Massage   88, 138
    Stress relieving tool   110
    Therapy, miracle solution   167
Mattress
    Healing bedding, miracle solution   167
Meditation   88, 108, 112, 118
    Miracle solution   167
    Stress relieving tool   102, 103–105
Memory loss   107, 153, 175
    Symptom of chronic illness   16

O

Obesity
    Standard American diet   49
    Trans fats and HFCS   63–65, 173
Ocular migraine
    Symptom of chronic illness   16
Oil pulling
    Miracle solution   167
Omega-3s   64, 174, 175
Organic   50, 144, 146-147, 174, 179
Osteoporosis
    Hormonal imbalance   162
Over the counter (OTC)   160, 174

P

Pain
    Archeologist   26-28
    Bone   79
    Burnoff overview   97–98
    Fibro trifecta   23
    Headaches   28
    Muscle fatigue
        Exercise   92–94
    Pain fade
        Burnoff   27, 97-98
    Pain sensitivity   22
    Pain varieties
        Sue's definition   26–28
    Widespread
        Symptom of chronic illness   16
Palate
    Re-education   51, 70, 151
Paresthesia   15
Peach paradigm. *See* **Emotional wellness**
Pesticides
    Environmental toxins   160
    Farm   3

R

S

T